R for XRNs

A Step-by-Step Guide to Manage Stress, Reduce Overwhelm, and Conquer Burnout

Terry Maluk, MSPH, RYT

Rx for RNs: A Step-by-Step Guide to Manage Stress, Reduce Overwhelm, and Conquer Burnout
© 2018 by Terry Maluk

ISBN: 978-1-7327729-0-8
Library of Congress Control Number: 2018910866

Printed in USA by Terry Maluk

Author photo on the back cover by Steve Cozart, Steve Cozart Photography.
Front cover images courtesy of 123RF.
Images on pages 37 and 64 courtesy of Adobe Stock.

The publisher has strived to be as accurate and complete as possible in the creation of this book.

This book is not intended for use as a source of health, medical, or financial advice. All readers are advised to seek services of competent professionals in the health, medical, and financial fields. Readers are cautioned to rely on their own judgment about their individual circumstances and to act accordingly.

For more information, visit http://FromStressedToCalm.com

For bulk book orders, contact
Terry Maluk
Terry@FromStressedToCalm.com

Dedication

For All the Nurses:

Dictionaries tell me you're "a person who is trained to care for sick or injured people." They have no idea. Thank you for your service, which goes far beyond words and definitions.

For Nurses Emmi, Sharon, and Craig:

Thank you for your unwavering love and support.

Table of Contents

Dedication iii

Acknowledgments. vii

Special Gift from Terry ix

Introduction. xi

Chapter 1:   The First Thing You Need To Know 1

Chapter 2:   Got Stress? 5

Chapter 3:   Breathing In Calm 11

Chapter 4:   There's Magic In Your Smile 25

Chapter 5:   Discover Clarity 33

Chapter 6:   Discover Your Tapping Genius 45

Chapter 7:   Discover Stealth Tapping .63

Chapter 8:   Discover Inner Peace 71

Chapter 9:   Discover Profound Rest 83

Chapter 10: Rediscover Your Brilliance 89

Chapter 11: Discover Confidence 99

Chapter 12: Go-To Stress-Relief Tools 109

Afterword 113

Notes. 115

Special Gift from Terry. 119

About the Author. 121

Acknowledgments

I celebrate my village of friends, family, and experts who have supported me throughout the writing, editing, publishing, and launching of this book.

Thank you, Wes, for being an amazing life partner, my travel buddy, my true companion.

To my daughter Sarah and my granddaughter Emmy, thank you for giving me instant reasons to smile each day. You are my heart.

To my friend Emmi Mooney, thank you for repeatedly helping me find the courage to do things out of my comfort zone.

Blessings and thanks to Molly MacCartney and Spirit, who inspired and guided me as I wrote this book.

Thank you, Book Shepherd Diana M. Needham, and your excellent team for helping make this dream a reality.

Special Gift from Terry

Now that you have your copy of *Rx for RNs*, you're on your way to recognizing and managing stress, overwhelm, and burnout. As you read this book, you'll understand the difference between good and bad stress, how chronic stress impacts your physical and emotional health, and you'll have an entire toolkit you can use to quickly and easily stop stress in its tracks. Plus, you'll learn easy ways to say "no" (even if you've never been able to before) and to set healthy boundaries with confidence.

As my gift, you'll also receive the special Relax, Tap, and Rest Kit that I created as a supplement to this book. This Kit includes:

- a quick seven-minute guided relaxation audio so you can relax even when you don't have much time,
- a concise "How to Tap" video that clearly demonstrates the Emotional Freedom Techniques (EFT) Tapping process, and
- a twenty-five-minute guided yoga nidra audio, which is an enjoyable way to feel fully rested.

Visit https://FromStressedToCalm.com/bookbonus/ to register for your Relax, Tap, and Rest Kit. You'll also receive stress management tips and information from me every few weeks. Your contact information will never be shared with anyone, and you can unsubscribe at any time.

The sooner you learn and practice using these simple tools for releasing stress, the sooner you'll start thinking, feeling, and sleeping better.

Here's to you . . . you've taken care of everyone and everything else. Now it's your turn.

All the Best,

Terry Maluk

Introduction

I'm so happy you've chosen this book to help you manage your stress and feelings of overwhelm. I know you'll enjoy learning and practicing these tools and discovering the freedom of less stress. This path is ultimately about self-care because that's what it takes. Before we begin, I'd like to share my story, so you know you're *not* alone. I've been where you are, and there *is* hope.

Mid-career, I began working in the technology field, helping to provide the public with online data and information about natural hazards. I truly loved my career. As part of a great team, we each had our strengths and learned from one another for an efficient redundancy of expertise. We enjoyed a sense of pride as we worked together to provide the best services possible.

I spent over fifteen years in that role and eventually became the team manager. During that time, organizational charts changed, management styles shifted, and budgets tightened. It was harder to get approval for needed resources, and upper management was becoming more removed from the reality of daily operations and less understanding of what it took to keep things running efficiently. "Do more with less" was the theme. What had always been rewarding became stressful. Looking back, I recognize this was when I started experiencing physical symptoms I didn't know were related to stress.

I let my work life intrude on my home and family life because I couldn't set healthy boundaries. Headaches became chronic migraines, low back pain started limiting my activities, and I was waking up at 2:00 a.m. worried about work.

Sound familiar?

The chronic stress of ever-changing priorities and demands was taking its toll on my body and my happiness. When I started having chest pains, my doctor gave me sobering news. I realized it was critical for me to find a way to relieve the constant stress.

So, I had a decision to make. I didn't want to quit, so I had no choice but to make some changes. I did the research and learned a variety of stress-relief techniques. At first, I worked on my own to relieve the physical pain, and then I found teachers and coaches who showed me exactly how to use time-honored and leading-edge techniques with quick and amazing success. They helped guide me to dig deeper into the underlying causes of my physical symptoms.

Relieving my pain by reducing chronic stress allowed me to get back to enjoying the things I love to do, like hiking in the mountains, traveling, and scuba diving. I even began sleeping better! Based on my experience, I was convinced these techniques could help others as well. And that is how my journey as a Stress-Relief Specialist began!

It took a couple years of trial and error as well as training and practice to discover the techniques that worked best for me. I customized my stress-relief toolbox with all the techniques that helped me reduce and manage my stress triggers both at work and in the rest of my life.

Why did I write a book specifically for nurses when I'm not a nurse myself? Because I *am* a member of the American Holistic Nurses Association and I believe nurses and caregivers need information about stress-management tools that work quickly and easily. Because my life has been blessed with family, friends, and clients who are nurses and I know what you're going through. Because I've spent months interviewing nurses about what you love about your career and what is taking you to the breaking point. Because you were there when my parents transitioned and that means the world to me. Because I don't want you to give up. You *can* save yourself and your career if you choose.

Research and evidence-based studies prove the tools in this book work to relieve stress. I began sharing with others what I had learned and to help them customize these techniques for themselves. I've guided many on the path to stress relief through talks, group workshops, and one-on-one sessions using a variety of tools that could be customized to meet their needs. I know these tools can help you, too.

The reality is that chronic stress will cause damage to your body and to your quality of life. The good news is you can do something about it. I'm honored to support you on this path.

I specialize in helping professionals like you relieve and reduce stress. By relieving the stress, we discover a cascade of benefits in our lives.

My qualifications include a Master of Science degree in Public Health and a Bachelor of Science degree in Science Education. I'm an accredited certified Emotional Freedom Techniques (EFT) Tapping Practitioner through the Association for the Advancement of Meridian Energy Techniques (AAMET). I have trained both through EFT Universe and through AAMET with trainers who worked directly with EFT founder Gary Craig. I'm a registered yoga teacher through Yoga Alliance and a certified Reiki master/teacher. I have also completed Matrix Reimprinting Training.

If you're ready to start letting go of your stress, you're in the right place!

Here's a little preview of our upcoming journey. This roadmap to managing stress and finding calm includes learning several techniques that are each proven to reduce stress in different ways and at different times. You'll be able to create your own stress-relief toolbox as you learn what works best for you in different situations, because one size doesn't fit all.

- An important part of stress management is learning to recognize how and when you begin to feel stressed. By practicing simple awareness, you'll begin to notice the first signs and be able to react quickly with a helpful tool. This will keep things from snowballing into stress at the first hint of a trigger.

- You'll learn several types of breathing you can use any time you start to tense up.

- You'll learn about the power of your smile.

- You'll strengthen your practice by celebrating wins. Research shows that by noticing and documenting our wins each day, and finding gratitude for each win, our level of happiness increases and leads to noticing more wins in our lives each day.

- You'll learn Emotional Freedom Techniques (EFT), also called Tapping, which will neutralize the negative emotions and physical reactions that accompany chronic stress.

- You'll experience relaxation meditations that will bring immediate calm and rest. You'll be guided through a twenty-five-minute yoga nidra session that will give you the benefits found in four hours of deep sleep! You'll be able to do this practice on your own anytime with the audio provided. (Relaxation meditation audios are included in the book bonus Relax, Tap, and Rest Kit created specifically for you. Visit https://FromStressedToCalm.com/bookbonus/ to download them.)

- With daily practice, you'll become comfortable enough with the tools that you'll soon notice a renewed sense of self-confidence. With that confidence and practice, you'll find it easier to start setting healthy boundaries at work and at home by learning easy ways to say "no." Many of us have trouble with saying this, so practice is good!

- You'll also get helpful hints on quick and easy go-to methods for stress relief.

Let's get started!

Terry Maluk

Terry@FromStressedToCalm.com

Please remember: It's important to contact a professional if things feel too big for you, whether it be a physician, psychologist, psychiatrist, or certified EFT practitioner. Never discontinue your current medications without first consulting your doctor.

Chapter 1

The First Thing You Need To Know

Does this sound like you? You've done the research and found a few tools to help reduce the stress in your life. You've read about how these methods work, listened to the audios and watched the videos (promising to practice them when you really need them). Now, you're waiting for a stressful situation so you can pull them out of the tool-box, right? You're ready to let go of all that stress!

Well, only reading about the methods and listening to the audios (but not practicing regularly) won't help you relieve stress. The first thing you need to know about destressing your life is this: you need to *commit to practicing* these methods at least once each day, *before a crisis*, so you become an overall calmer person who no longer reacts in the same old ways when the proverbial $&@% hits the fan. The good news is that practicing isn't hard. And, with practice comes progress toward a calmer and happier you. That's your goal, right? You *can* do this!

Nurses tend to be caregivers by nature. Nurturing, altruistic, and compassionate, nurses can be selfless to the point of self-neglect. It's ironic that while nurses have a crucial role in taking care of everyone else, nurses often put their self-care last. Over time, this leads to exhaustion, feelings of overwhelm, and burnout, which helps no one.

The nonstop demands in the environments where most nurses work may not always support self-care. Sometimes it's even hard to take time for a bladder break! But it's important to take self-care seriously if you want to continue being of service in such a high-stress profession.

Honoring basic needs such as taking the time to use the restroom as needed so you're not afraid of staying hydrated, having time to enjoy a healthy meal or snack, and taking periodic breaks to pause, take a slow breath, and regroup should be the norm, not the exception. Committing to a daily practice of the stress-relief techniques in this book will help you continue to be your best self both at work and at home.

Let's talk about what happens when stress strikes. Imagine your supervisor unexpectedly asks if the task you were given is on schedule and you know it's not. Maybe the census is ridiculous, and you just learned that your day or night will be short-staffed, meaning your shift will be a nightmare. What's your reaction? If you're like most, your heart rate increases, your digestion slows, your immune system is weakened, and your thinking, creative brain goes offline. You go into fight, flight, or freeze in reaction to the stress. Your body releases stress hormones to deal with the perceived threat, which is a normal reaction that's meant to protect you.

But while you're in that state, your responses and answers might not be the best. Your ability to think and make a quick decision is hampered, adding further stress. This is hardly the time to pull out a new tool to try to relieve stress even if you could remember those tools at that stressful moment. And when stressful situations happen daily, you're awash in the stress hormones, which takes a toll on your physical and emotional well-being. So, what can you do?

You can commit to learn and practice your tools early and often, *at least once each day, starting today*. With regular practice, a few tools will soon become second nature and start automatically in stressful situations because you've given your body new ways to help self-regulate your reactions. I've had many clients report this new auto-response to stress.

Other tools, when practiced regularly, help make you more resilient and less reactive to stressful situations overall, so the fight, flight, or freeze reaction doesn't get the chance to kick in. Because you're now more aware, you remain calmer, more confident, and more in control of the situation—no matter what gets thrown at you. Your typical reactions are replaced with more effective ones, which takes rehearsal! Don't wait until you're facing a terrible situation to practice stress relief techniques. Be prepared in advance so that when the time comes, you're ready!

I highly recommend you begin with the seven-minute guided relaxation audio bonus from my website (https://FromStressedToCalm.com/bookbonus/).

It will guide you to a calmer state and is the quickest and easiest way for to you start right now. For this audio to be helpful, you need to *choose* to listen to it all the way through with patience and courage. To eliminate distractions, find a quiet, comfortable place and give yourself the gift of starting this journey with one small seven-minute step.

I believe in you.

JOURNALING YOUR EXPERIENCE

Describe how you feel today about starting this journey. What emotions are you feeling? Do you feel those emotions in your body? Take a moment to notice your feelings and record them below. There are no right or wrong answers.

_____

_____

_____

_____

_____

_____

_____

_____

_____

_____

_____

_____

_____

_____

_____

_____

_____

_____

_____

_____

_____

_____

_____

_____

_____

_____

_____

Chapter 2

Got Stress?

Does any of this sound familiar? You wake up exhausted. Your mind races thinking of all the things you need to do today. You're in a constant rush to get somewhere and to get everything done because there's never enough time. You give up on your to-do list and just try to make it through the newest crisis at work or at home. There's no time to fix a healthy meal, so fast-food takeout or pizza delivery is the easiest choice. And of course you feel guilty about that, so why not have the cookies, too? Running errands in heavy traffic on the way home leaves you overwhelmed and frustrated. The chores at home are building up. And then the washer breaks. Really?! By the time the day is done, you're exhausted, but you decide to check your email. Then you can't fall asleep, or you wake up in the middle of the night, going over all the things that went wrong that day. When the alarm goes off, you wake up exhausted. . . .

Sadly, this situation is all too familiar for a growing number of people. Stress has become an expected part of life. When I speak to groups, I'll ask for a show of hands from those who are feeling stressed. Almost every single person raises their hand, nodding their head in understanding. Sometimes we wear our stress like a badge of honor and compare stories about how much of it we have in our lives. I know I've participated in conversations like that in the past.

So, what exactly is stress? The American Institute of Stress defines it this way: "The term 'stress,' as it is currently used was coined by Hans Selye in 1936, who defined it as 'the non-specific response of the body to any demand for change.' Through experimentation, Selye found that short-term stressful situations can result in impacts on the stomach, lymph system, and adrenals. He found that chronic or long-term stress can result in heart and/or kidney disease, stroke, and rheumatoid arthritis. He later defined stress as 'the rate of wear and tear on the body.'" [1] Selye's research attracted much attention and *stress* became a well-used buzzword to describe many situations.

There can be good stress (eustress), such as winning an award, being offered an exciting new job, getting engaged to be married, or buying a house. But stress is most often identified with things that aren't so good (distress): bills, relationship problems, or the boss from you-know-where.

Some say that a little stress in life is good to help with performance. Nothing like a call from an upset supervisor to motivate you, right? Others disagree, saying any amount of stress is bad. But either way, when you're stressed, you definitely don't do your best creative thinking. When your body is in fight, flight, or freeze mode because of perceived threats, you aren't at your best for making good choices quickly. Can you imagine doing a math problem while being chased by a tiger? While a looming deadline at work isn't a tiger, your body perceives that deadline as a threat, taking your creative brain offline because you're impacted by the stress hormones.

It's been shown that remembering or retelling a stressful event from the past causes the body to react as though it were happening again. It's clear that stress management has become a necessity for many people to avoid health issues, prolonged illness, and insomnia. Chronic stress, day in and day out, at work and at home, is not a good thing. So, it's crucial that you recognize your warning signs and limit how much stress you're exposed to and your reaction to it.

When you sense perceived danger of any type, your body begins to produce stress hormones. Three major stress hormones include adrenaline, norepinephrine, and cortisol. Adrenaline and norepinephrine help you to focus on the threat, allowing you to become more aware of and awake to it. Your heart and breathing rates increase, your muscles tense, you may even start sweating. Blood flow shifts from less critical areas, like digestion and analytical thinking, to your muscles so you can react physically—run—if you need to. You're on high alert to react to the perceived threat.

The amygdala, the alarm center of the brain, makes a decision based on previous experience to determine whether a situation is a threat. For example, the last time the boss called an emergency meeting with the team, someone was unexpectedly fired, and you immediately start worrying that you may be next. But once the situation is perceived as non-threatening, the all-clear signal is given. Your body begins to return to a resting state, which can take anywhere from thirty minutes to a few days.

If the situation *is* perceived as dangerous, a cascade of signals to other parts of the brain and body produce more chemical reactions, which ultimately result in the production of the stress hormone cortisol, secreted by the adrenal glands. This response is perfect to help you get out of a dangerous situation quickly and efficiently. It's meant to get you through the crisis, after which you can shake it off and get back to a resting state.[2] However, when you live in a state of chronic stress, you stew in stress hormones. You never get a chance to return to a normal rest and digest state.

The body's reactions to this stress soup include elevated cortisol levels that interfere with your learning and memory; compromised immune function; reduced bone density; increased weight; higher blood pressure and cholesterol; and increased risk for heart disease. You can also experience blood sugar fluctuations and get sick more often. Aches and pains increase. Elevated levels of cortisol, if unchecked, increase abdominal fat, which is associated with heart attacks and strokes. Studies show that chronic stress and elevated cortisol also increase the risk for depression, mental illness, and can lower life expectancy. These chemicals and the feelings they create can also be addictive. So, while stress isn't good for you, it can leave you wanting another "hit" because you unknowingly crave it.

One of my clients was struggling with making lasting progress on relieving her stress. As we worked together, we made sure she could feel the results of each tool. She agreed to practice, and she experienced some great results. And then her practice time would decrease until she stopped entirely. What caused her to give up once she started seeing the results of reduced stress? Her body was rebelling because it was addicted to the rush of stress hormones and the familiar feelings she was so used to having. Once this concept registered with her, we practiced techniques to address this unconscious self-sabotage trick. She became aware of her reactions and choices, and she started practicing her tools again with great success.

All this is scary stuff, and you don't want to get stressed out about being stressed out. So, what do you do when you see warning signs, or worse yet, miss the warning signs and reach a breaking point, like I did? Thankfully, there are many helpful methods to reduce stress.

In this book, you'll learn about these methods, techniques, and tools, and how to use them. You'll have quick success with some tools, while others will work for the long term. All of them will help to one degree or another in different scenarios. As I mentioned in the first chapter, if you want these tools to work, you must commit to practice them. To successfully apply them takes an awareness of your feelings and reactions, which you may have become numb to.

Ready? I know you can do this. You *are* strong enough!

Journaling Your Experience

What would life be like for you without all the stress and overwhelm?
Describe how that would feel.

_____

_____

_____

_____

_____

_____

_____

_____

_____

_____

_____

_____

_____

_____

_____

_____

_____

_____

_____

_____

_____

_____

_____

_____

_____

_____

Chapter 3

Breathing In Calm

You have this amazing relaxation tool with you everywhere you go: your breathing. Most of the time, you probably don't even notice it. Breathing just happens automatically, thankfully, and you can go about your business. Or is that busy-ness? You may find you stay so busy that you forget to take a moment or two to just stop, *be still, and breathe*. It's such a simple act, yet not always so easy to do. It can be hard to remember to stop what you're doing and take a breath. Being still for a moment will give you the chance to regroup.

Yet, you may resist stopping to take care of yourself because you have so much to do. How can you possibly stop? "I don't have time to stop and be still! Are you kidding me? What about my patients, this work-load, these tasks, the kids, my partner, the laundry, the house, the dog, the bills . . . I could go on and on!"

Do you find yourself telling stories of how stressed you are to anyone who will listen? Do you wear the badge of stress proudly? Do you compare stories with friends and colleagues about just how bad things are? Do you tell your stories repeatedly? Did you know that each time you share a story, you're reliving the stress? Your body jumps on the stress hormone roller coaster as it tries to protect you from this threat, even when the threat isn't present in this moment. Maybe it's time to stop telling your stories, refocus, and start reducing your stress.

The weight of feeling overwhelmed and stressed can sit on your head, in your neck, and in your shoulders, weighing you down emotionally. When you feel it increasing, you might think you need to move faster and do more. But, when you're stressed, your body feels threatened by something it can't deal with. So, it's important to reduce your stress levels every chance you get. One quick and easy way to do that is to stop and take a breath with complete awareness. In other words, turn your full and complete attention to the simple task of breathing.

There is so much about breathing to notice. In one breath, you become aware of the temperature of the air being inhaled. On the next, you notice how far you feel the air move into your body. In the next breath, you see if the chest or belly expands as you inhale. As you exhale, you notice that everything releases.

You can intentionally make the breath longer and deeper. Focus on the tip of your nose and take in and release a few very slow, comfortably deep breaths. (In all these breath awareness techniques, make sure to breathe slowly enough, so you don't feel light-headed.) Then return to normal breathing and notice how you feel. How long did that take? Maybe two minutes? Is it worth it? My experience has been that I always feel better after even a single mindful breath. You're now ready to learn a few breathing methods to help you discover calm.

THE CALMING POWER OF BREATHING

Research shows that mindful breathing activates the body's natural relaxation response. Breathing is the number one way to quickly and easily release, relieve, and reduce stress. And by practicing mindful breathing, you'll begin to more easily recognize and take advantage of the opportunities to practice throughout the day.

Mindful breathing is a powerful stress reduction tool because it helps you feel better right away! There are many ways to use breathing to relax. This first one is a simple method that's easy to learn and remember, works quickly, and can be practiced anywhere, anytime. As with every technique in this book, familiarize yourself with it first by reading through the steps before diving in.

- Find a place to sit or recline comfortably. Be still. You can close your eyes if the situation and your comfort level allow. You can practice wherever you are, even standing or walking down the hall.

- Begin to notice your natural breathing pattern. Your mind will begin to settle down when you give it something to focus on.
- Then on your next inhalation, say to yourself, "Inhaling."
- And on your exhalation, say to yourself, "Exhaling."
- Continue as time allows.

Now it's your turn. Breathe at your own comfortable pace. For this practice, there's no need to force the breath to be faster or slower, longer or shorter. Just breathe. When you notice your mind starting to wander (and it will), gently bring it back to focus on your breathing. Start with five breaths.

> Exhale completely, and begin . . .
>
> *Inhaling. Exhaling.*
>
> *Inhaling. Exhaling.* (Notice where you feel your breath in your body.)
>
> *Inhaling. Exhaling.*
>
> *Inhaling. Exhaling.* (Notice your thoughts. Gently bring them back if they've wandered.)
>
> *Inhaling. Exhaling.*

Repeat if you'd like to practice that again. If you're ready to add to the practice, you can introduce a reminder to *relax*. As you breathe in, say, "Inhaling. Relax." As you breathe out, say, "Exhaling. Relax." As you say the word "Relax," notice if there's any tension in your body. Focus on where you feel tension and consciously try to loosen and relax the muscles in that area. Most people hold tension in their shoulders or their jaw. Notice where you're holding tension and try to let it go. Practice now for five breaths.

> *Inhaling. Relax. Exhaling. Relax.*
>
> *Inhaling. Relax. Exhaling. Relax.*
>
> *Inhaling. Relax. Exhaling. Relax.* (Notice any tension in your body and try to let it go.)

Inhaling. Relax. Exhaling. Relax.
Inhaling. Relax. Exhaling. Relax.

How do you feel now? Do you find it's getting easier to focus on your breathing? Did your mind wander a bit? It's normal and natural for your mind to do that. The fact that you noticed your mind wandering means you're becoming more aware of what's happening in your body. Each time you notice your mind has wandered:

- Recognize that it's happened,
- Release the distracting thought,
- Notice any tension and relax that area of your body,
- *Smile* to celebrate that you noticed, because that's a big step,
- And then start your breathing practice again.

Here's a little hint: If you find your mind constantly wandering as you practice, try counting your breaths. As you breathe in, say to yourself, "Inhaling 1" and as you breathe out, say to yourself, "Exhaling 1." Then "Inhaling 2, Exhaling 2," and so on. Continue counting until you reach 10. If your mind wanders again, gently start over at 1. No self-criticism. No judgment. Just breathe. I promise this gets easier quickly.

I'm frequently asked how deeply you should breathe during this exercise. As long as you're comfortable and not forcing the breath but simply noticing it, you're doing it correctly. If you choose to deepen and lengthen the breath while practicing, that's fine too. You can include this change in your practice by saying to yourself: "Inhaling deeply. Exhaling deeply." Again, being comfortable is important, especially when you're first starting this practice.

Another question I'm asked is whether participants must sit in a special position. No, you can do this anywhere, anytime. If you prefer, you can rest back in a reclined position. You might fall asleep, though, so set a timer if you need to. And you can use this breathing technique intentionally to help you fall asleep. While many practitioners use a special upright seated posture with the legs crossed, the perfect position for you is the one you're in when you need calming breaths. Enjoy this quick and easy breathing practice to help you relax and find calm anytime you need it.

Three More Breathing Techniques

As I mentioned, nothing is easier than simple mindful breathing for reducing stress. Below are three more breathing techniques that really work. And I know they can work for you, too! Test them all. Notice which ones become your go-to breathing methods in times of stress and begin building your personal stress-relief toolbox!

Heart Breathing

If you want to quickly collect your thoughts, feel calm, and be more fully present, try using *heart breathing*. Heart breathing is an easy method of releasing stress and bringing you back to your center. Below is a summary of the step-by-step instructions based on the description from the HeartMath Institute for using the technique. Enjoy!

- Read through the instructions first, so you know what you'll be doing, then get comfortable. If you like you can close your eyes while you breathe.
- When first learning this technique, put one or both hands over your heart to more easily bring your attention to that physical area. (Once you know how to do this, there is no need to move your hands to your heart, which makes it easier to do anywhere and anytime.)
- Let your breathing be natural and just a little deeper than normal.
- Imagine you're breathing directly into your heart center, and then exhaling from your heart center. This gets easier with practice.
- Now begin to count as you inhale and exhale. Breath into your heart center comfortably to a count of six. Then breathe out from your heart center to a count of six. Adjust your counting pace to match your unique breathing pattern.

- Continue inhaling and exhaling to a count of six as you focus on your heart center.
- Notice a sense of calm and peace settling in as your focus shifts to your heart.
- Repeat as needed.

It's as simple as that. I like to take *at least five or six breaths* like this, but spend as much time as you like practicing. You can use heart breathing anytime. It's great first thing in the morning and again as you close your eyes to sleep at night. Try it when you get a stressful email or phone call, when you're in traffic, before or during a meeting or a test, and any time you just want to feel calm, centered, and relaxed. There are no negative side-effects, and you can do it as often as you like. With increased awareness of the heart center, you will also find yourself feeling more open in that area and feeling more joy for life.

Abdominal Breathing

You may notice when you're stressed you take quick, shallow breaths, which robs your body of the benefits that a full breath provides. Learning to use abdominal breathing means breathing fully from your abdomen (the bottom of your lungs) near the diaphragm. By taking intentionally slow, comfortably deep breaths, you reduce stress and its negative impacts on your body.

The American Institute of Stress provides an excellent breathing technique that allows your relaxation response to settle in quickly and easily. You can use it anywhere, and it's easy to do: just take ten slow, comfortably deep abdominal breaths following the instructions below.

Begin by noticing your current breathing.

- Are you breathing rapidly or slowly?
- Are your breaths shallow or deep?
- Where do you feel your breath in your body?
- Where do you feel expansion in your body when you breathe in?

Now, move into abdominal breathing.

- Place one hand on your abdomen right beneath your rib cage.
- Take a slow, comfortably deep breath in through your nose, breathing all the way into the bottom of your lungs.
- Your chest may rise slightly, but your stomach should rise noticeably, and it should push your hand up and out.
- When you see your hand moving up and out as you inhale, you know you've got it.
- Pause for just a moment with a full breath, and then exhale *slowly and fully through your mouth.* Control your exhale, so it lasts longer than your inhale.
- As you exhale, try to release and let go, relaxing all the muscles in your body.
- To allow the relaxation response to settle in, make sure to take at least ten abdominal breaths.
- Keep the breaths very slow and smooth to keep from getting dizzy.

The American Institute of Stress recommends twenty to thirty minutes of abdominal breathing each day but *start with ten breaths* and build up as time and your comfort level allow.

Ocean-Sounding Breath

This technique feels a little funny to do at first. Adults are usually self-conscious about trying it. When I teach a children's yoga class, I tell them if they sound like Darth Vader, they're doing it right. This gives them a chance to laugh and feel less self-conscious and provides a reference they know and will remember! While the text suggests you sit or recline, once you know how to do this type of breathing, you can do it anywhere and anytime. Try it and see how it works best for you.

- Find a comfortable place to stand, sit, or recline where you won't be disturbed. If you're reclining, support your head with something soft, and you may wish to place a pillow under your knees so that your spine can completely relax. Take a moment to get comfortable. Settle in. Make any adjustments you need so you're completely relaxed.

- Scan your body and notice any areas of tension or tightness and try to relax them. Allow your eyes to close if that's comfortable for you. Notice your natural breathing. Notice the length of your inhalation and exhalation. Breathe normally; don't try to force the breath in any way. Simply notice.

- After a few normal breaths, begin to *slowly deepen and lengthen each breath*, taking in a little more air on your next inhalation. Allow your exhalation to be more complete, fully emptying the lungs. On your next inhalation, breathe in a little deeper and notice your lungs expanding a little more. Your next exhalation is more complete, emptying all the air out of your lungs. Very slow, comfortably deep breaths. Inhaling. And exhaling.

- Now *let your jaw relax* enough so that your mouth gently opens. As you exhale through an open mouth, make the sound of fogging up a mirror or your sunglasses, *haaaaah*. Notice the slight constriction in your throat. Maintain that as you inhale, so you make the same sound. Continue inhaling. And exhaling.

- Make sure your breathing is slow and deep enough, so you don't feel light-headed.

- *Notice your thoughts*. If they have wandered, gently bring them back to focus on your breathing. Give yourself the gift of being fully present, open to full relaxation, right here, right now.

- Continue with your slow, steady breaths, making the sound of gentle ocean waves.

- With practice, once you feel confident in this style of breathing, you may want to *try closing your mouth but maintaining the slight constriction* in your throat. Your ocean waves are quieter, but you can still hear them.

- Release your deep breathing after *five to ten breaths* and allow your breath to come back to its normal pace. Let your eyes slowly blink open. Notice how you feel.

Use this simple ocean-sounding breathing style to bring calm and relaxation whenever you need it. With practice, you'll notice additional benefits such as increased lung capacity and increased self-awareness.

The first time I ever attended a yoga class, it was at the mature age of fifty-two and at the encouragement of a good friend. I was fortunate to find a studio that focuses on breathing, which solidified my decision to return for a second class versus giving it up entirely. As a distance runner, my flexibility left much to be desired, so I needed the stretching. But the breathing!

After a particularly long and stressful work day, trying to finish up a conference call on the drive to the yoga studio, I felt my energy and self-confidence take a dive. And here I was, doing something new in an unfamiliar place surrounded by strangers. But in that one-hour class, as I learned to practice the ocean-sounding breath, I was transformed. I couldn't believe how relaxed I felt. The seven minutes of resting at the end of the class, where you lie still, breathing normally, and the teacher brings you a pillow and a blanket if you want, clinched it. This experience might have had something to do with why I became a registered yoga teacher. It meant I could bring the gift of relaxation to others, which has become my passion.

You've learned several ways to use your breathing to bring calm. It can be as simple as a deep sigh, or as involved as you like. But each of these techniques can be used exactly when appropriate and as needed. Remember that *daily practice* lecture I gave earlier? That's your homework. Choose at least one of these breathing techniques and practice each day. You'll thank me later. I promise.

For more information on how breathing helps you feel calmer and more relaxed, see the Notes section at the end of this book.[1, 2, 3, 4]

Journaling Your Experience

Take a moment now to write about your experiences with each of these breathing techniques.

How did it feel as you began to focus on your inhalations and exhalations? Is this focus new for you?

_____

_____

_____

_____

_____

_____

_____

_____

_____

_____

_____

What was your experience as you practiced the heart breathing?

_____

_____

_____

_____

_____

_____

_____

_____

_____

_____

_____

Where and when can you see yourself using this practice?

_____

_____

_____

_____

_____

_____

_____

_____

_____

_____

_____

If you have practiced heart breathing in a real-time situation, how did it work for you? Can you think of a way to customize heart breathing for yourself?

_____

_____

_____

_____

_____

_____

_____

_____

_____

_____

_____

_____

What was your experience using the abdominal breathing?

_____

_____

_____

_____

_____

_____

_____

_____

_____

_____

_____

Where and when can you see yourself using this practice?

_____

_____

_____

_____

_____

_____

_____

_____

_____

_____

_____

_____

_____

If you have practiced abdominal breathing in a real-time situation, how did it work for you? Can you think of a way to customize abdominal breathing for yourself?

_____

_____

_____

_____

_____

_____

_____

_____

_____

_____

_____

_____

What was your experience using the ocean-sounding breath?

_____

_____

_____

_____

_____

_____

_____

_____

_____

_____

_____

_____

Where and when can you see yourself using this practice?

_____

_____

_____

_____

_____

_____

_____

_____

_____

_____

_____

If you have practiced the ocean-sounding breath in a real-time situation, how did it work for you? Can you think of a way to customize the ocean-sounding breath for yourself?

_____

_____

_____

_____

_____

_____

_____

_____

_____

_____

_____

_____

_____

Chapter 4

There's Magic In Your Smile

Did you know research has shown that the simple act of *smiling* can lift your mood and reduce stress? Psychoneuroimmunology, the study of how the brain is connected to the immune system, has also shown that happiness boosts the immune system. When you smile, the brain interprets the muscle activity as an "all is well" message, signaling the release of feel-good chemicals, including dopamine, which makes you feel happier, and serotonin, which is associated with reduced stress.

Even better, merely activating the facial muscles as you smile, even if you're faking it, has the same effect. Your brain can't tell the difference. So, you can use the "fake it 'til you make it" approach until your smile is genuine. Usually, this doesn't take long.

But sometimes stress is so extreme that even faking a smile isn't possible. This is where you can use the old "one-two" approach to breaking the cycle of stress. First choose your favorite breathing technique from Chapter 3 and practice it for one to five breaths. Doing this first will then help your face ease into a smile, even if it's fake!

One of my clients insisted that she couldn't smile during a specific, extremely stressful situation. "Nope. I just can't do it," she said. As our session continued, we worked on using the heart breathing technique. She imagined inhaling "calm" directly into her heart and letting it float up to the top of her head. She then exhaled as she imagined that calm feeling cascading down from her head, surrounding her body in a bubble of peace. After the third breath like this, she suddenly exclaimed, "Now I can smile!" Try the heart breathing technique if you just can't find your smile.

When you're tense, your muscles tighten, including your facial muscles. You may find you're clenching your jaw when you're stressed. Smiling can help release a little of that stress by quickly relaxing your face. How easily do you smile? Are you always able to find a quick, genuine smile during your day? Or does it take effort sometimes? Have you noticed a difference in how you feel when you allow yourself to break into a smile? Smiling is a great resource you can use when you're experiencing a rough spot in your day. Smile all the time. Be aware of what your face is doing more often and make an effort to smile every chance you get.

Another way to easily find your smile is to offer someone a compliment about something. You can offer a cashier a compliment on their hair or nail color, tell a co-worker you like their shirt or shoes, thank your partner for something they did. The possibilities are endless. After you do that, watch their face. Most often, they'll look into your eyes and then smile. Notice how that makes you feel. In that instance, finding your own smile will be almost automatic.

Your smile can be contagious. Notice how others react when you smile. Maybe their face softens a bit and they smile too, reducing *everyone's* stress. When you make eye contact with and smile at someone, notice how the look on their face changes. They'll most likely smile back because you've taken a moment to recognize them and offer kindness through a smile. They may think about how it made them feel. Maybe they'll take up the practice of smiling at others to warm their hearts as well. I love smiling while I'm driving. It's quick, easy, and free!

CELEBRATE THE GOOD

Sometimes you may find yourself so overwhelmed with everything demanding your immediate attention that it's impossible to see the small positive things in your day. What if you could also give your attention to the good things? What if you tried to recognize and acknowledge the good in your day, the wins as they happen, and then take a moment to smile and celebrate them? It might just turn the day around from overwhelm to merely controlled chaos, right? This fun mood-lightening process takes only a few minutes each day and will help open your eyes to all that is good.

Even if you're stressed to the bone, you can find a reason to celebrate. There's always someone or something you can recall or notice around you that can be seen as a win, such as…

- The weather is great!
- The supervisor heard and agreed with something you suggested!
- Your team is fully present and focused!
- You may have an entire afternoon without a meeting!
- The power bill is lower than you expected! (It could happen!)
- The traffic wasn't too bad, and somebody let you merge with a smile!

You get the idea. Take a moment and put in a little effort to notice something positive. You can even say an enthusiastic "Yes!" out loud, or air high five if that makes you feel good. And if you just can't get to a place of celebration or gratitude at that moment, try a few slow, comfortably deep breaths first to unfreeze and relax a little.

Here's the thing: you can take the practice of celebration a big step further by writing down a few wins each day. It's surprising how this small effort really works to reduce stress and calm the mind and body. When you feel good and celebrate those wins, you'll begin to notice more good things each day. It's all about awareness.

Of course, there's the flip side. When you don't feel good and only notice the negative, you tend to focus on that, making it feel like there are only conflicts and stress in your life. So . . . you *can* make the choice to help yourself feel better about your day!

Being Grateful

Dedicate a journal or notebook in which you can record your daily wins. Use an electronic journal if that works for you. Because I travel so often, I switched from my paper journal to an electronic version on my phone, and it works great.

- If you're using a physical notebook, you can give it a title. If you're creative, draw something on the cover or tape a relevant image there. If you're using an electronic version, import images and design it to reflect your style if you like.

- Start by putting today's date on the first page.

- Write or type your first win entries! Try to find at least three wins each day. These can be one-word wins or paragraphs explaining each win scenario: who was there and what happened in as much detail as you want. You can use images, artwork, whatever it takes for you to celebrate and smile.

- Do this again tomorrow, and the next day, and the next. Be as consistent as you can. Like all the tools in this book, this gets much easier the more you do it. I always look forward to this daily practice.

- If you miss a day, don't quit. Just start again. Starting again is your win: "I started to celebrate again!". *attitude of gratitude*

Not surprisingly, research shows that finding gratitude each day can improve physical and psychological health, reduce stress, reduce aggression, increase empathy, improve self-esteem, and increase resilience. And you'll especially love this benefit: a 2011 study showed that when participants spent a few minutes each evening writing down or typing out the things for which they were grateful, it helped them to sleep better and longer! If you're like me, when you sleep well, you feel better. And then you smile more and see and express gratitude more readily. Everything is, indeed, all connected.

An Easy Challenge That Can Make A Difference

Here's a challenge for the next time you're pulling up or walking in to your workspace. Instead of approaching it with a negative mindset, anticipating walking into a situation you dread, see if you can notice *one thing* to celebrate. It can be anything, big or small. Hints if you need them: good weather; a good parking space; the smell of fresh coffee; the sunrise or sunset colors; someone else's smile; a kind gesture by someone in traffic; no wait time for the elevator; clean restrooms; flowers in the workspace; a brand-new day; the sound of laughter; remembering you have choices; and your ability to take a mindful breath. I know you can find them, and I promise it gets easier the more you practice. If you do this consistently, you'll notice a shift in how you show up in your workspace.

Small changes in your daily habits can make a big difference. If you keep showing up in the same way, doing the same things day in and day out, you can't expect things to get better. But with daily practice, letting go of old habits that keep you stuck, and choosing new ones that will help you reduce your stress, you can change your life for the better!

JOURNALING YOUR EXPERIENCE

Take a moment now to write down the names of a few people who make you smile easily. Then think about things in life that give you a reason to smile and write those down, too. The more you practice this, the more reasons you'll find to smile. It's a win-win. Refer back to this list anytime you need a smile.

_____

_____

_____

_____

_____

_____

_____

_____

_____

_____

_____

_____

_____

_____

_____

_____

_____

_____

_____

_____

_____

_____

_____

_____

When you begin to notice that you can choose to smile more easily during your day-to-day situations to help relieve the stress, this is a huge victory! Awareness of your choice is a big step. And when you choose to smile during your day-to-day situations to help relieve the stress, how does that make you feel?

_____

_____

_____

_____

_____

_____

_____

_____

_____

_____

_____

_____

_____

_____

_____

_____

_____

_____

_____

_____

_____

_____

_____

Chapter 5

Discover Clarity

First let's check in with your breathing, smiling, and celebrating wins practice. How is the breathing work going? Have you used it in a real-time stressful situation yet? Were you able to write down and celebrate your wins each day? Are you starting to notice a change in your overall stress level? I hope you're starting to see what's working best for you as you build your stress-relief toolbox. Your favorite tools will change over time as you learn new techniques. You'll find some tools work in certain situations better than others. For now, notice what works for you and trust you can reach for your best tools any time you need them.

In this chapter, you'll learn to decode your top stress triggers with a simple, yet profoundly powerful technique that's scientifically proven to reduce stress and anxiety. By learning to focus on exactly what is stressing you, and how it's affecting you, you gain clarity and the ability to laser focus on the issue and release the stress more easily. Sound too good to be true? It's absolutely true and has been proven to work by scientists and those who practice it worldwide. Worried that this will never work for you? You've got nothing to lose and so much to gain by making a commitment to try it for yourself.

INTRODUCTION TO EMOTIONAL FREEDOM TECHNIQUES

Emotional Freedom Techniques, also called EFT Tapping, or just Tapping, is a simple, straightforward method to help you reduce stress that can provide relief in minutes. One of the things I love about EFT Tapping is that it's a self-help tool. You can use EFT Tapping to reduce stress whenever you need to, and it will help you recognize and clear any resistance you might have to creating a more calm, peaceful, and rewarding life.

A Little History in a Nutshell

EFT uses gentle tapping on some of the same energy lines or meridians used in acupuncture and acupressure, combined with the current psychology technique of talk therapy (Cognitive Behavioral Therapy).

The work of psychiatrist Dr. John Diamond, chiropractor Dr. George Goodheart, and psychologist Dr. Roger Callahan led to a surprising discovery in the 1970s. Their patients experienced relief for a variety of issues including fears, phobias, and stress by talking about their problems while stimulating certain energy lines. Callahan patented the technique calling it Thought Field Therapy (TFT). TFT was one of the first methods developed in the field of what is now called Energy Psychology.

Gary Craig, a Stanford-trained engineer, was interested in the field of personal development and studied the work of Dr. Callahan. As Craig realized the potential of this approach, he worked to refine and simplify TFT techniques while maintaining positive, measurable results: an evidence-based methodology. He ultimately developed a simple and effective set of techniques he called EFT, which he made available to everyone on his website in the 1990s.[1]

Since then, EFT has continued to undergo testing and refinement by many individuals and groups. Publications in highly respected, peer-reviewed journals continue to support Craig's findings and techniques. Craig's Gold Standard EFT is considered to be the original or classic version of EFT.

Groups such as the Association for the Advancement of Meridian Energy Techniques (AAMET International), EFT Universe, National Emotional Freedom Techniques Training Institute (NeftTI), and others have developed EFT training and certification options for those interested in pursuing the use of this tool to help themselves and others.

How Tapping Works

As discussed in an earlier chapter, when you experience or even remember something stressful, the fight, flight, or freeze alarm goes off in your brain. In an efficient cascade of physiological responses, that alarm causes stress hormones to be produced that help you fight, run, or freeze to avoid danger. Usually the perceived danger doesn't warrant a full-out alarm response. Often it's just a memory. But your body reacts as though it was happening in the present moment. The result is that you're frequently exposed to stress hormones unnecessarily. And that's not good.

When stress hormones are circulating in your system, they slow or stop digestion, compromise your rational thinking, and reduce the effectiveness of your immune system. When you live in a chronically stressed condition, you can expect to see physical and emotional consequences.

And this is where EFT Tapping comes in.

Gentle stimulation via tapping on specific points on your hand, head, and torso sends a calming signal to the alarm center in the brain that all is well, even though the threatening thought is still present. The specific points used in EFT coincide with known acupuncture points on your body's energy lines. The understanding is that tapping on these points disrupts and removes energy blockages and releases stress from your body's energy system, which encompasses the body's energy lines. As Craig discovered, "The cause of all negative emotions is a disruption in the body's energy system."[2] With repeated tapping, your brain finally gets the message: this thing that was previously filed as "dangerous" isn't a threat. Your energy balance is restored, and you return to a healthier state both physically and emotionally.

The Basic Recipe

The easiest way to learn how to tap is to use the Basic Recipe, which includes the specific tapping points on the body and the different statements said while tapping. It also includes making an estimate of the intensity of your physical or emotional discomfort, so levels can be compared before and after tapping to measure progress. It might sound complex, but it's very simple.

Once you've practiced EFT Tapping even a little, you'll more easily find your own words to match what you're feeling, which will be most beneficial to you. It's very important to use words that describe *specifically* what you're feeling and where you're feeling it in your body to get the quickest and most long-lasting results.

Let's take this step-by-step with a simple example.

1. First, *focus on an issue* that's bothering you right now. It could be physical or emotional. Be as specific as you can with your description. For this example, we'll be focusing on a specific stressful event: "That stressful argument I had with my supervisor in the hallway on Tuesday."

2. Next, *estimate the intensity level* of the stress you're feeling about that event or issue on a scale from 0 to 10, where 0 is no stress at all and 10 is maximum stress. I recommend you write your number down for later comparison to check your progress. I'll tell you a quick story later about why that's a good idea.

3. The *setup statement* is where you acknowledge the problem and then state that you accept yourself anyway. You tap on the *side of the hand point* while saying the setup statement. That's the fleshy area between the base of the little finger and the top of the wrist on the side of the hand. You can tap on either hand. I like to tap with all four fingertips of the opposite hand, but you can use one or two fingers. While gently tapping the side of the hand point, repeat your setup statement three times. For example: "Even though I had that stressful argument with my supervisor in the hallway on Tuesday, I accept myself anyway." *Repeat the setup statement three times* while continuously tapping on the *side of the hand* (SH) point. Refer to the EFT Tapping Points image for the location of all the points used in the Basic Recipe.

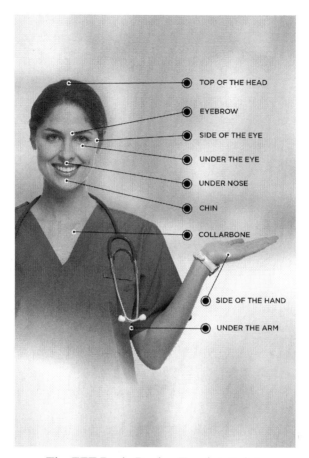

The EFT Basic Recipe Tapping Points

4. After the setup statement, tap on the *other eight tapping points* shown in the image. With your fingertips or a flat hand, gently tap about seven times on each of the other points while saying the *reminder phrase*: a few words or a brief phrase that reminds you of the problem. For example: "That stressful argument with my supervisor." The number of times you tap isn't critical, so don't worry about counting them. Just tap and talk.

5. Start tapping gently on the *top of the head point* while saying your reminder phrase: "That stressful argument with my supervisor."

6. Continue to the next point which is the *eyebrow point*, on the inner edge of the eyebrow, right where the eyebrow starts near the bridge of your nose. You can tap either or both eyebrow points with one or two fingers. Tap gently while saying your reminder phrase: "That stressful argument with my supervisor."

7. Next, tap gently on the bone at the *side of the eye*, either or both eyes, while saying your reminder phrase: "That stressful argument with my supervisor."

8. Then follow the bone around and tap gently *under the eye* (either or both), while saying your reminder phrase: "That stressful argument with my supervisor."

9. Now tap just *under the nose* above the top lip while saying your reminder phrase: "That stressful argument with my supervisor."

10. Next, tap on the *chin point*, which is in the crease under your bottom lip and above your chin, while saying your reminder phrase: "That stressful argument with my supervisor."

11. Then find the v-notch at the base of your *collarbone*. Move down and out about an inch or so to find the slight indentations there. You can tap either or both sides. I like to gently tap the whole area with an open hand. Tap there while saying your reminder phrase: "That stressful argument with my supervisor."

12. Finally, tap about four inches *under the arm* on the side body, either or both sides, while saying your reminder phrase: "That stressful argument with my supervisor."

You've completed one round of tapping. I know it seems like a lot to remember when you're first learning, but I promise it quickly becomes second nature after only a few rounds of practice. After tapping on all those points, *take a slow breath* and *notice your intensity level again* on a scale from 0 to 10. Write it down next to the original number for comparison.

You don't need to worry about getting this exactly right. With practice you'll know what is right for you.

Once you're familiar and comfortable with the steps of the Basic Recipe, you might notice you want to tap longer on one spot than the others. That's fine to do. Follow your instincts about what's right for you. You can keep saying the same reminder phrase at each point, or you can change it as thoughts or words come to you; however, keep your focus on what's bothering you for the first rounds. You aren't going to reinforce the negative thoughts and emotions by saying them. Instead of continuing to ignore them, you're acknowledging them while you are signaling to your body you're safe and that it's OK to release them.

If your intensity level is still above 5, continue tapping more rounds until you get it down to as close to 0 as possible. Ask yourself what's keeping it above a 0 and then tap on that!

Know that as you tap your mind relaxes. Old memories may come to the surface, or sudden insights on why you're feeling a certain way may appear. Keep your notebook handy to jot things down so you can tap on them later. Or, if the memory is more intense than what you're currently working on, you may want to switch over to tapping on that memory and finish up what you had originally started tapping on later.

What if I Can't Say I Accept Myself?

Remember the setup statement you use when you start the Basic Recipe? It has two parts. As EFT founder Gary Craig describes them, the first part includes your acknowledgment of the specific problem. The second part affirms your acceptance of yourself despite the problem: "I deeply and completely accept myself." How does it feel to say that out loud? Does it feel true?

If you have no problem with those words, continue using them as long as they feel comfortable and true for you. You may want to look at the other options below just in case you encounter a situation that causes you to feel less comfortable stating your self-acceptance.

You might be so worked up about an issue it's hard to say those words out loud, and it might be hard to feel they're true. Maybe it's always hard to say them. If so, try something a little different. Consider these options: "Even though I have all this stress,"

> "I'm open to someday accepting myself."
>
> "I'm willing to consider accepting myself."
>
> "I accept my feelings, and I'm OK."
>
> "I can someday accept myself without judgment."
>
> "It might be safe to accept myself."
>
> "I choose to try to accept myself."
>
> "I accept how I feel."
>
> "I'm willing to accept myself."
>
> "I allow myself to accept myself."
>
> "I'm OK!"
>
> "Even though I have a hard time saying I accept myself, I accept myself anyway."

Jedi mind trick, the last one is.

You have many options to choose from, depending on how you're feeling. Give yourself permission to create your own options. The goal is to reach the point where you can say something positive at the end of your setup statement. As you keep saying it, perhaps it will eventually sink in as truth in your heart. At least try to be open to that possibility! (And breathe. This is a great time to practice breathing in feelings of calm and self-acceptance.)

Everyone has weaknesses and limitations. Some days, you might not be willing to state out loud your self-acceptance. But if you try first using EFT Tapping on the general feeling of not accepting yourself, you may relieve a bit of the panic and distress and may calm yourself enough to do more specific tapping work. I call that progress!

There are so many helpful videos and websites with tapping scripts available. You may find even stronger positive acceptance statements including "I deeply and completely love and accept myself." If you can say that, awesome! If not, substitute with a positive affirmation that's true for you.

Why Should I Write Things Down?

I mentioned earlier to make a note of your initial and ending intensity during each tapping practice. It's also a good idea to write down the issue or emotion, feeling, or sensation you're tapping for. Here's why.

In a private coaching session, one of my clients had a very intense issue to work through. As we talked briefly about the issue, I took notes of her words to use for her specific setup statement and reminder statements. I noted how she felt because using specific words is what gets the best results. I then asked her what her level of intensity about that issue was. She replied, "Oh, it's a 10!" She had no doubt about that intensity, so I wrote that down as the starting point.

Because her intensity was a 10, we started tapping on the general feeling she was having before going deeper and using her specific words. It took three rounds using her specific words until I could see a change in her face and body posture that signaled she was releasing the negative emotion. She even yawned, which is a great sign of release that you will likely experience as well. After we finished those rounds, I checked in with her about her intensity level. Her words were, "Well it's a 0. It really wasn't bothering me that much to begin with." I showed her my notes where she reported it was a definite 10, and she was surprised.

I explained to her that as she taps, she's able to relax, and a change in her body and mind occurs, which releases the negative, stuck energy. Once that energy is released, she's no longer holding on to the stress or intensity of the event and may even think it was never stressful to begin with. I've experienced this myself, so I'm always glad to have the proof of my initial intensity, which I always write down before I start tapping. So, remember to write down your intensity levels before and after so you can measure your EFT Tapping success!

A QUICK SUMMARY

Can you see the potential for using EFT Tapping to get beyond the stress and overwhelm? Tapping can be used for everything!

Here is a summary of the Basic Recipe steps:

1. Identify the issue.
2. Write down the initial intensity level 0 to 10.
3. Say your setup statement three times while tapping on the *side of the hand.*
4. Say your reminder statements while tapping at the other eight points.
5. Guess your new intensity level and write it next to your initial intensity level.
6. Repeat tapping with the same or new words until the intensity is down to 0 or as close as you can get. (There are several advanced EFT Tapping techniques to deal with stubborn issues.)

I hope you will allow yourself time to practice EFT Tapping daily and keep a journal of your results. Start with five minutes each day and practice for as long and as often as you want. Use the Basic Recipe for guidance as needed. If you get stuck, tap without words and see what happens! You'll find this new tool pays off in big ways.

Also, continue with your breathing, smiling, and celebrating wins practice. Using these tools in combination with EFT Tapping makes them even more powerful. Now you have more tools to help you go from stressed to calm and reduce the feelings of overwhelm.

In the next chapter I'll give you a few simple scripts you can use while you're learning to tap and searching for your own words.

JOURNALING YOUR EXPERIENCE

Write down your first impressions of using EFT Tapping so you can look back on them later. You'll be amazed at how quickly you gain confidence using this technique.

_____

_____

_____

_____

_____

_____

_____

_____

_____

_____

_____

_____

_____

_____

_____

_____

_____

_____

_____

_____

_____

_____

_____

_____

_____

_____

As you become familiar with the different tapping points, notice if you prefer to tap on one or more of the points longer than the others. And if you do, describe your experience.

_____

_____

_____

_____

_____

_____

_____

_____

_____

_____

_____

_____

What is your current favorite affirmation at the end of your setup statement? Revisit this over time to see if it changes.

_____

_____

_____

_____

_____

_____

_____

_____

_____

_____

_____

_____

Chapter 6

Discover Your Tapping Genius

While my clients are first learning EFT Tapping, one of their most frequent questions is "What do I say while I tap?" At first, you may know how you feel but be at a loss for words and afraid that you're doing it wrong. Tapping scripts give you the comfort of knowing you're saying something relevant, but you don't have to come up with the words by yourself. Tapping scripts can be helpful at the start of your EFT Tapping practice. Below are scripts that deal with some common stress-related issues. You'll be able to go from Newbie to Tapping Genius quickly!

USING TAPPING SCRIPTS

While the use of tapping scripts is common in the world of EFT Tapping, the opinions on the use of scripts are many! Some certified EFT practitioners discourage the use of scripts because you aren't using your own specific words. The concern is that pre-written scripts may be too generic for the user to realize real and lasting results.

Other practitioners encourage the use of scripts, so you have a good foundation from which to explore. While I'm providing a few scripts for you to learn the basics of EFT Tapping, I *highly* encourage you to substitute the words in the scripts with your own words as soon as possible. In this way, you'll more quickly learn to trust yourself during your EFT Tapping sessions. The scripts are kind of like training wheels—don't get dependent on them. Trust yourself to find your words.

Migraine Relief Script

One of the most common stress-related issues that my clients experience is headaches, often full-blown migraines. Migraine headaches are always painful and sometimes completely debilitating. Many migraine sufferers spend several days unable to work or even stay in an upright position. Migraines can return often, effectively stealing your precious time and robbing you of happiness.

Sometimes the cause can be physical, such as when you become dehydrated. Often the cause is chronic stress or a past trauma you continue to play out in your mind, causing an emotional blockage and disruption in your body's energy. EFT Tapping is proven to help reduce and eliminate physical pain and clear emotional blockages. Therefore, EFT Tapping can help relieve and even eliminate migraine headaches. My personal experience using EFT for migraines has proven to me it works amazingly well.

I have the type of migraines that produce a visual pattern warning about ten minutes before the pain and nausea strike. I've learned that if I start tapping as soon as I get that visual warning, I'm able to keep the migraine from becoming full-blown. Many of my clients who are nurses have chronic headaches and migraines. If you, too, suffer from headaches and migraines, you can first address the *physical pain* using the following example setup and reminder statements. Please use the specific wording that applies to your headache as soon as you're ready.

Ask yourself a few questions to help find your words:

- What are you feeling in your body? Where is the pain, exactly?
- Does the pain have a color?
- How big is it: small like a marble, or big like a beach ball?
- Does it have a texture: smooth, scratchy, sharp?
- Is it hot or cold?
- Is it constant, throbbing, intermittent, or something else?

Yes, it really is helpful to get *that* specific, because you'll use these words in your setup statement and in your reminder phrases. You might not have an answer to all those questions, but ask yourself the questions anyway.

Next, guess at the intensity level of your headache pain on a scale of 0 to 10, with 0 being no pain, and 10 being the worst you can imagine. Write that number down in your notebook for later comparison. (Refer to the Basic Recipe and image in the previous chapter if you need a reminder of the location of the tapping points.)

Repeat your setup statement three times, using words that describe how you feel, while tapping on the *side of the hand* point. For example:

> "Even though I have this sharp, red pain about the size of a basketball from this migraine headache, I completely accept myself."
>
> "Even though my head feels like it's splitting and it makes me feel nausea in my stomach, I completely accept myself."
>
> "Even though I have this sharp, red pain from this migraine, I completely accept myself."

Then move through the other tapping points. Tap especially gently on the points on the top of your head and your face, with reminder statements that describe exactly how you feel. For example:

> *Top of the Head (TOH)*: "This sharp, red pain in my head."
>
> *Eyebrow (EB)*: "This migraine headache."
>
> *Side of the Eye (SE)*: "This nausea in my stomach and this sharp, red pain in my head."
>
> *Under the Eye (UE)*: "I really don't have time for this migraine right now."
>
> *Under the Nose (UN)*: "This awful pain in my head."
>
> *Chin (Ch)*: "It feels like a tight band around my head."
>
> *Collar Bone (CB)*: "I feel terrible."
>
> *Under the Arm (UA)*: "I'm so tired of this headache."

After one or more rounds of tapping, take a slow breath, and guess again at the intensity level of your pain. Write it down next to your original number. Maybe the number has gone down significantly. But if not, continue gently tapping to reduce the intensity level even more.

Tapping on the *side of the hand*, repeat this setup statement three times:

> "Even though I still have some remaining headache pain, I accept myself anyway."
>
> "Even though my head still hurts a little, I completely accept myself."
>
> "Even though I still have some remaining headache pain, I accept myself anyway."

Continue to the other tapping points and describe how your head and body feel:

> *TOH*: "This remaining headache."
>
> *EB*: "And I'm still a little nauseous."
>
> *SE*: "This remaining headache."
>
> *UE*: "This remaining nausea."
>
> *UN*: "This remaining headache."
>
> *Ch*: "I'm ready to let this headache and nausea go."
>
> *CB*: "I'm ready to release this headache."
>
> *UA*: "It's safe to release this pain now."

If the number isn't going down after repeated rounds, it may not be purely a physical issue. It may be time to look at possible *emotional* causes. Did any thoughts or memories surface while you were tapping? Is there is an emotion that comes up (overwhelm, fear, anger, frustration, etc.,) when you think about your headache? You can then tap about the specific emotion you're feeling. Your setup statement might sound like this: "Even though I feel all this anger in my chest right now, I accept myself and how I feel."

You may have an idea of what brought on your migraine, such as a stressful work situation, a family argument, or some other recent event. You can then tap specifically on that situation or event. Your setup statement could sound like this: "Even though this _____ issue is really stressful for me right now, I completely accept myself." Fill in the blank to describe the situation or issue that is bothering you.

If you don't have a clue about what emotions might be behind this thumper of a headache, your setup statement could be: "Even though I just don't know, I completely accept myself anyway."

When tapping on the "I don't know" statement, you may experience memories or insights that lead directly to the source of your emotional upset. Then you can tap on that. Like the layers of an onion, you will slowly peel each one away until you've discovered the core issue(s) that you can then neutralize one at a time using EFT.

Your body is usually trying to protect you as it goes into its fight, flight, or freeze routine. What happens when you've been working way too many hours for too long, not getting enough sleep, not eating right, and getting no physical exercise? Eventually, your body will take charge and *create* a reason for you to slow down, such as a migraine or other physical pain or illness. Can you think of a time in the past when that might have happened to you?

It's important not to rebel against or be angry at your body when this happens. Instead, try using words that show gratitude and understanding in your tapping:

> "Even though I have this migraine and it hurts too bad to work right now, I appreciate my body for trying to protect and help me take care of myself."
>
> "Even though I have this pain, I understand that my body is just trying to protect me, and I'm OK."
>
> "Even though I have this pain, I hear my body loud and clear and I'll find a way to slow down and release the pain."

I've used this approach for my migraines, and it works like a charm!

Back Pain Script

Another common physical symptom of chronic stress is back pain, most often in the lower back. This physical issue can be approached in the same manner as you would for headaches, using descriptive words in your setup statement and reminder phrases that describe exactly what you're feeling and where. Remember to ask yourself questions to help you find specific words:

- What are you feeling in your body? Where is the pain exactly?
- Does the pain have a color?
- How big is it: small like a marble, or big like a beach ball?
- Does it have a texture: smooth, scratchy, sharp?
- Is it hot or cold?
- Is it constant, throbbing, intermittent, or something else?
- Include other questions that might help describe what you're feeling.

Rate the intensity level of the pain on a scale from 0 to 10 and write that down in your notebook. Then start tapping! Below is a script with suggestions for words you can use as a starting point. Change my words to your words as soon as it feels right for you. Take a breath and trust yourself.

Tapping on the *side of the hand*, repeat your setup statement three times:

> "Even though I have this constant, burning hot, sharp pain in my lower back on the left side, I accept myself anyway."
>
> "Even though I have this constant, burning hot, sharp pain in my lower back on the left side, I accept myself anyway."
>
> "Even though I have this constant, burning hot, sharp pain in my lower back on the left side, I accept myself anyway."

Move to the other tapping points and describe how your pain feels:

> *TOH*: "This constant, burning hot, sharp pain in my lower back on the left side."
>
> *EB*: "This constant, burning hot, sharp pain in my lower back on the left side."

SE: "This constant, burning hot, sharp pain in my lower back on the left side."

UE: "This constant, burning hot, sharp pain in my lower back on the left side."

UN: "This constant, burning hot, sharp pain in my lower back on the left side."

Ch: "This constant, burning hot, sharp pain in my lower back on the left side."

CB: "This constant, burning hot, sharp pain in my lower back on the left side."

UA: "This constant, burning hot, sharp pain in my lower back on the left side."

Notice I used the exact same words in the setup statement all three times, and the exact same reminder phrase each time. This is an easy method that works well, too! If you have trouble finding other words, just use the same ones for each point. It's not a requirement to change the words each time.

After one or more rounds of tapping, take a slow breath and guess the intensity level of your pain. Write it down next to your original number. Did anything else come up as you were tapping? Look for any emotions or events that may be related to the pain and use tapping to clear those to help clear the pain. Lather, rinse, and repeat.

Are you starting to see the pattern now? Next you can practice while focusing on the feeling of overwhelm that you might experience.

Reduce the Overwhelm Script

With overwhelm, you may often feel buried in tasks, by a never-ending to-do list, with real and perceived time constraints, under pressure from multiple sources including yourself, and with a recurring theme of *"too much!"*

When feelings of overwhelm begin to surface, remember to start your breathing practice right away to keep yourself present and calm enough to remember to tap. It might seem like just another thing on your to-do list, but by tapping, you become more efficient in your thoughts, and you'll save time in the long run. As I mentioned earlier, rather than waiting for the overwhelm to get the upper hand, a short daily tapping practice can make all the difference.

In this chapter, you've been refining your EFT Tapping practice from general tapping to tapping for exactly what you're experiencing. But overwhelm can be much broader than specific physical pain because the overwhelm may be coming from multiple sources and directions. To begin, start by noticing, acknowledging, and working to calm the immediate sensations that come with overwhelm.

On a scale of 0 to 10, with 0 being not overwhelmed at all and 10 being completely overwhelmed, how intense is your feeling of over-whelm at this moment? Write it in your notebook and start with simple tapping. If you're at a 10, I recommend you begin by tapping without words on all the points for a few rounds so you can find your words.

If you're ready to tap with words, try being emphatic when saying them so you convey the emotions you are feeling.

Tapping on the *side of the hand*:

> "Even though I feel so overwhelmed, I accept myself anyway."
>
> "Even though I feel so overwhelmed, I accept myself anyway."
>
> "Even though I feel so overwhelmed, I accept myself anyway."

One simple reminder phrase on the other tapping points:

> *TOH*: "I feel so overwhelmed."
>
> *EB*: "I feel so overwhelmed."
>
> *SE*: "I feel so overwhelmed."
>
> *UE*: "I feel so overwhelmed."

UN: "I feel so overwhelmed."

Ch: "I feel so overwhelmed."

CB: "I feel so overwhelmed."

UA: "I feel so overwhelmed."

Write down your intensity level next to your original number. Notice if your number has changed. If the number is the same, continue with the general tapping statements. If the number has gone down a bit, you can ask yourself questions to see what comes up for you, so you can become more specific:

- As you think about the feeling of overwhelm that you have, what is the first thing that comes to mind?
- Is it a particular project or deadline?
- Is it bills or financial issues?
- Is it a co-worker or other relationship issue?
- Is it an exhausted and hopeless feeling?

Once you identify a single issue to work on, estimate your intensity level about that single issue and begin tapping on the *side of the hand*. (I'm using "this project" in the example, but substitute your own words when you're ready.)

"Even though I feel exhausted because of this project, I completely accept myself anyway."

"Even though I'll never get it all done, I accept myself anyway."

"Even though there is too much to do and not enough time, I completely accept myself."

TOH: "I am so exhausted."

EB: "There is just too much to do."

SE: "And not enough time."

UE: "And there's not enough me!"

UN: "This just stresses me out."

Ch: "I feel so overwhelmed."

CB: "I can't even think straight."

UA: "Everything is just swirling in my head."

Continue straight into a second round by going right back to the top of the head.

TOH: "Why can't I ever get a break?!"

EB: "Why can't I just finish this project and move on?"

SE: "I'm doing the best I can."

UE: "But it never seems to be enough."

UN: "And then I get frustrated with myself and everyone around me."

Ch: "I just want to stop the chaos in my head."

CB: "So I can think better."

UA: "Maybe then I'll be able to prioritize things."

And now a third round! You have so got this!

TOH: "I wonder if it's possible,"

EB: "That I can do what needs to be done once I feel calmer."

SE: "And I know I'll feel calmer if I can just take care of myself."

UE: "Maybe it's OK to stop and breathe and tap from time to time."

UN: "I know that I think better after I take the time to breathe and tap."

Ch: "I'm doing the best I can do right now."

CB: "And I choose to take care of myself."

UA: "I choose to feel more calm and relaxed so I can be my best self."

Take a slow breath and estimate the intensity level you feel about that single issue after those three rounds. Write it down next to your first number. You can tap as many rounds as necessary to start to feel better. Each round takes so little time; you can do amazing things in as little as five to ten minutes. How do you feel? Were you able to substitute more specific words about how overwhelm feels to you?

Once your intensity levels are as low as possible, a three or below, you can begin to insert positive statements into your EFT Tapping! But it's important to tap down the negative intensity before you do that. Otherwise, it's like sweeping it under the rug again.

Positive statements might be:

"I'm starting to feel better already."

"I know I can handle these tasks."

"And I choose to slow down enough to help organize my thoughts."

"I know this will all work out once I can think straight again."

"And I'm thankful that I remembered how to tap and breathe so I can find calm again!"

We covered a good amount of tapping in this chapter. Try not to get too bogged down in the details at first. Just tap, with or without words.

Case Studies

So that you understand the depth of stress and strength of EFT Tapping, I want to share two case studies from clients with whom I've worked. These are amazing people just like you who were able to take the same tools that are presented in this book and use them to create more freedom and joy in their lives. They have less fear and fewer cravings. They're more radiant and confident. It all started with their commitment to self-care.

Anna

Anna (not her real name) is a nurse who was suffering from overwhelm while working in an acute care facility full-time, going to school part-time, and trying to keep up with her family demands. Stress came from all directions: she felt chronically exhausted, she was worried about her growing debt from tuition, she wanted to spend more time with her son but shift work didn't always make that possible, and she had an important exam coming up. Anna started experiencing trouble sleeping and having nightmares about taking the exam.

While Anna had been holding it together for two years under a chronic stress load, the upcoming exam was the last straw. All the buried and blocked emotions and negative energy started coming up: fear of failure, fear of spending all that tuition money for nothing, fear of losing her job if she didn't finish this degree, guilt for not spending more time with her family, and overall frustration and exhaustion.

As we worked together, Anna learned breathing techniques that she used often. She learned to recognize the tightness in her chest that started when she thought about the exam, and she used breathing techniques to relax the tightness, which kept it from spiraling into panic. She learned EFT Tapping to address her fears of taking the exam and possibly failing it. Using calming tools like breathing and tapping helped her focus better so she could study more effectively. The nightmares stopped almost immediately.

We used heart breathing and tapping while visualizing the exam scenario until she could walk through the whole process in her mind comfortably with a smile on her face. She stopped waking up in the middle of the night panicked about the exam.

Anna learned confidence-building tools that allowed her to see herself in a new way. She felt calm and confident as she approached exam day, breathing and tapping multiple times each day to keep her center of calm.

Anna reported to me right after she took the exam and learned her score. She didn't lose her confidence as she began the exam, and she practiced her slow, calming breaths throughout. She even used a Stealth Technique that you'll learn in Chapter 7 twice during the exam when she needed a little extra reassurance. She passed with flying colors and now has a toolbox she can use for all her upcoming exams. Passing her exam was a big win she celebrated and noted in her journal.

Anna's fear of failing exams is gone. (She finished her degree!) Related fears have disappeared as well with continued breathing and tapping. We continued to work together to release some other issues that came up, and she is now using these self-help tools regularly to confidently deal with any remaining day-to-day stress as it arises.

Julia

Stress can show up in so many ways. Julia came to me to work on a common stress-related issue for caregivers: food cravings. She was gaining weight and felt powerless to do anything about it. She felt frustrated because she had no control over her eating at home, which tended to happen after working her 12-hour shifts, saying, "I just lose control."

Using EFT Tapping is a quick and powerful way to reduce and eliminate food cravings. Julia liked the idea that tapping could help her regain control over her eating. I reminded her that we're not trying to deprive ourselves and that we aren't saying that we can never have that food again. It's all about taking back our control by reducing the triggers.

I asked Julia to bring to the session the "go-to" food that she craved the most and had the most trouble resisting. She brought a Snickers bar, one of my favorites too. We reviewed the tapping basics, and then I asked her to think about when she shops for Snickers and the sound of the wrapper when she opens it. Next I had her open the Snickers and smell it. Julia estimated her craving intensity at that moment at "about an 8 or 9." So we started tapping right away.

After a few rounds, I asked Julia to smell the Snickers bar again. She looked surprised and took another sniff, then told me that it didn't smell the same as before. I told her she could take a small bite, which she did. She made a face and said it didn't taste like she remembered. She even put the Snickers bar down and pushed it away! These are very common reactions. The good news is that EFT Tapping really does work that quickly to reduce and eliminate a food craving.

The full story is that tapping once for a food craving isn't a complete solution. Cravings are often the result of some blocked emotion. With regular tapping, we can uncover and release these blocked emotions and get to the cause of the cravings. In Julia's case, it was all about the stress of her nursing job, the long hours often without a proper meal which caused low blood sugar and poor food choices, and the feeling of being deprived and exhausted when she got home.

Julia was trying to make herself feel better with her favorite quick treat. By recognizing that pattern, she chose to plan meals to take to work, to bring a healthy snack to enjoy in the car on the way home, and to practice tapping for the craving when she didn't want to indulge. She was then free to choose to indulge in moderation when it felt right to her. EFT Tapping helped Julia begin practicing self-care in a balanced way so that her weight gain stopped!

Remember: It's important to contact a professional if things feel too big for you, whether it be a physician, psychologist, psychiatrist, or certified EFT coach. Never discontinue your current medications without first consulting your doctor.

JOURNALING YOUR EXPERIENCE

Now that you've had a chance to practice EFT Tapping for specific stress-related issues, what questions do you have? (You can even ask them on the Facebook page: https://www.facebook.com/FromStressedToCalm/)

_____

_____

_____

_____

_____

_____

_____

_____

_____

_____

Are you becoming more comfortable finding your own words in your tapping practice? What makes it easier for you to find your specific words?

_____

_____

_____

_____

_____

_____

_____

_____

_____

_____

Tapping often prompts memories or insights during a session and sometimes even hours or days later. Do you experience memories or insights into the feelings and emotions behind your tapping topic? Describe that experience and how it helps you find clarity to release the negative energy.

_____

_____

_____

_____

_____

_____

_____

_____

_____

_____

_____

_____

_____

_____

_____

_____

_____

_____

_____

_____

_____

_____

_____

_____

_____

_____

_____

_____

Have you noticed that sometimes your body will try to protect you by creating an excuse for you to avoid doing something you'd rather not do? Awareness of this possibility is key. Describe an example of when that may have happened to you. How will your increased awareness help you avoid similar issues in the future?

_____

_____

_____

_____

_____

_____

_____

_____

_____

_____

_____

_____

_____

_____

_____

_____

_____

_____

_____

_____

_____

_____

_____

_____

_____

_____

_____

One of the most frequent comments my clients say is: "This probably has nothing to do with it but. . . ." You'll likely experience these seemingly random and unconnected thoughts after a round or two of tapping, and it's important to explore them. Have you experienced this yet? Did it lead to an "Aha" moment for you? Describe your experience here.

_____

_____

_____

_____

_____

_____

_____

_____

_____

_____

_____

_____

_____

_____

_____

_____

_____

_____

_____

_____

_____

_____

_____

_____

Chapter 7

Discover Stealth Tapping

Now that you're comfortable with using the Basic Recipe for EFT Tapping on different issues, it's time to learn two subtle Stealth Tapping techniques you can use just about anywhere.

TAPPING ON THE FINGER POINTS

Finger points are additional tapping points that can be added to the Basic Recipe when you encounter stubborn issues or they can be used alone. Because they can be tapped discreetly, you can use the finger points to tap anywhere or anytime, even if you aren't tapping on all the other points. Finger tapping can be an effective method of easily creating a beneficial daily habit of tapping.

Finger point tapping is convenient if you feel uncomfortable being seen tapping on all the other points, such as in a meeting or while you're out for a walk or run. This Stealth Technique is also useful when you're having trouble falling asleep or having trouble getting back to sleep. Rather than moving around too much while tapping on all the points, a gentle tapping on the fingers yields good results. With practice, you can even learn to tap on the finger points with the thumb or other fingers of the same hand, minimizing movement. Try it! There were times I used this method in one of my 2:00 a.m. sleep-interrupts and couldn't remember getting to all the finger points before falling back to sleep.

The tapping points on the fingers coincide with the same meridian lines located on the face and upper torso. They're in the same relative location on the thumb and three of the fingers, as shown in the

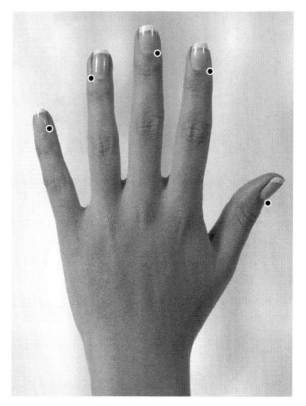

EFT Tapping Finger Points

image, which is at the side of the base of the nail. You may see other diagrams of the finger points that either skip the ring finger entirely or show the ring finger point on the same side as the other fingers. This consistency makes it easier to remember and practice. You can tap on either side of the ring finger, but since the energy line runs down the side where the point is shown in the image, I usually tap on the opposite side or sometimes even both sides of the ring finger.

Remember that EFT Tapping is a very forgiving technique, so there's no need to worry about getting it exactly right. Follow your intuition and practice what works best for you. The goal is just to tap. Experience the calm and relaxation that the simple Stealth Technique of finger tapping can provide you.

Hold and Breathe

When you really need to tap to relieve stress, but you don't feel comfortable tapping in front of others, use this even more Stealth Tapping technique!

Remember that EFT stands for Emotional Freedom Techniques. Notice that's plural because there are quite a few of these amazing techniques we can use. This simple method accesses the same energy lines we tap on in the EFT Basic Recipe, but allow you to do so much more discretely.

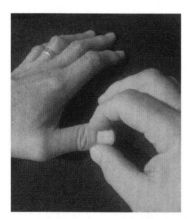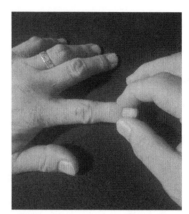

Hold and Breathe Points

My favorite Stealth Technique is to gently hold the thumb and then each finger in turn, as seen in the images above. Most often, this is done by using the thumb and index finger of the dominant hand to hold and gently squeeze both sides of the thumb and each finger near the corners of the nail bed on the other hand. Each finger is held for about as long as it takes for one natural breath cycle: one inhalation and one exhalation. Then move to the next finger.

Hold and Breathe is an inconspicuous method of using meridian endpoint stimulation to calm and release stress. You can do this in a roomful of people, and no one will notice. You can rest your hands in your lap or under a conference table during a meeting, and nobody will see what you're doing. You can use this technique standing in the hallway talking about a project with your hands casually behind your back or even in front of you. The possibilities are many, and the results are all good! I use this technique often to take the edge off as soon as I notice the warning signs that my stress level is climbing. This subtle technique can also be used when you find yourself awake in the middle of the night. Gentle pressure on the energy lines of the fingers allows you to feel calmer and to relax quickly so you can get back to sleep.

Because both finger point tapping and hold and breathe are Stealth Techniques, you don't need to vocalize anything while doing them unless you want to. Or you can say the words to yourself in your mind. You'll experience the benefits of neutralizing negative energy and dissolving blockages either way. Find what works for you and practice often.

Add these Stealth Techniques to the stress-relief toolbox you're building. Combine them with breathing, smiling, and celebrating wins for even better results on the road to a calmer, more relaxed you.

BONUS: HOW TO BE THE CALM IN THE STORM

In earlier chapters, you learned powerful tools to help you maintain a sense of inner calm regardless of what is going on around you. With these tools, you're at an advantage in any challenging situation. When you can keep yourself from entering the fight, flight, or freeze state, you're able to keep your best decision-making and thinking skills online. You'll do your best work if you can keep your head even when those around you are losing theirs. A quick shot of adrenaline can help prepare and motivate you to act, but drowning in it is what you're working to avoid.

When an unexpected crisis arises, you now know how to recognize your early warning signs of stress and panic. As soon as you're aware of the crisis, go into *Operation Calm* mode, so you're operating as your best self.

1. Use the easiest tool at your disposal first: *Breathe!*

   Consciously slow your breathing so that your body doesn't start the panic process, thereby giving you time to let your thinking brain calmly assess the situation and set priorities. Use any of the breathing techniques you've learned to regain and remain calm.

2. *Tap!*

   If you're in a situation where you can use the Basic Recipe for Tapping comfortably, go for it. Notice:

   a. How you're feeling,

   b. Where you're feeling it, and

   c. How intense the feeling is on a scale of 0 to 10.

   Tap using words that describe each aspect of your feelings for at least one round. Take a slow breath and repeat as needed and as you are able.

3. If you're in a situation that doesn't allow for the entire Basic Recipe Tapping, use a *Stealth Technique!* Remember to either tap on or gently hold the ends of your thumb and each finger. You can do this at the same time as you begin your breathing. Hold each finger for a full inhalation and exhalation and then move to the next one. Repeat as needed and as long as you're able.

Once you recognize the beginning of a stress reaction, and then find and maintain a sense of calm, control, and focus in the midst of a crisis, you'll be able to handle any situation that comes at you with confidence. And by consistently being the calm in the storm, you're setting an example for all those around you. Breathe. Tap. Focus. Share the Calm.

JOURNALING YOUR EXPERIENCE

Describe your experience using the two Stealth Techniques. Do you
have a favorite? Where might these techniques work best for you?

_____

_____

_____

_____

_____

_____

_____

_____

_____

_____

_____

_____

_____

_____

_____

_____

_____

_____

_____

_____

_____

_____

_____

_____

_____

_____

Are you becoming aware of how you feel when the first hint of stress starts taking hold? What are your favorite tools to use when you notice that feeling?

_____

_____

_____

_____

_____

_____

_____

_____

_____

_____

_____

Are you able to go into Operation Calm mode more easily now? Have you noticed if it helps those around you find a calmer state? Describe what you've experienced.

_____

_____

_____

_____

_____

_____

_____

_____

_____

_____

_____

Chapter 8

Discover Inner Peace

You've been working hard the past few chapters, learning new techniques that require you to do something to feel better. In this chapter you'll experience guided relaxation as a way to slow down and restore calm.

GUIDED RELAXATION

One of the easiest ways to discover inner peace and calm is to be guided through step-by-step instructions to reach a state of relaxation. For example, you can listen to an audio recording where your only task is to listen and allow relaxation to happen. Many guided relaxation audios include quiet background music or other calming sounds while others have only a gentle, soothing voice.

By treating yourself to guided relaxation recordings, you begin to increase your awareness of yourself, your environment, and your reactions. You'll experience the sense of peace that comes with releasing the stress of daily life in that moment. With regular use, you'll learn to more easily recognize your reactions to stress so you can better control them and gain confidence in your ability to manage stress at any time.

You can make this practice a special gift to yourself by making it a scheduled appointment on your calendar. I highly recommend that you set aside time where you won't be disturbed, so there's nothing else you need to be doing and nowhere else you need to be. In this way, you'll fully experience the benefits of guided relaxation.

If you haven't already, sign up at https://FromStressedToCalm.com/bookbonus/ to receive your free Relax, Tap, and Rest Kit, which includes a guided relaxation audio to help you find calm in less than seven minutes. Becoming still and listening to a guided relaxation audio is also an easy way to unwind and release the stress of the day.

MINDFULNESS MEDITATION

This chapter intentionally began with the introduction of guided *relaxation*, a widely accepted concept. When I began teaching yoga and meditation in a small community, occasionally a student would express discomfort with the word meditation as well as with the use of some of the traditional Sanskrit names for the yoga poses. For this reason, the teachers at the studio chose to use terminology that was more widely accepted in the region, as I've done in this book up to this point. But now it's time to dig a little deeper and talk about things like mindfulness, awareness, and meditation, all of which are practices that can help you go within to find and maintain a calmer state.

Meditation has been practiced in parts of the world for thousands of years. While archeologists and scholars agree that it has been practiced for about five thousand years, written records about meditation were discovered around 1500 BCE. It wasn't until the 18th century that translations began to make their way to Western scholars.

Many books have been written about various forms of meditation and how the practice has evolved over time; however, until recently, it was considered too "out there" in many people's minds to be seriously considered. Enter well-known authors such as Wayne Dyer, Deepak Chopra, Eckhart Tolle, Jon Kabat-Zinn, and many others, to help Western minds better understand the idea that a meditation practice can greatly improve the quality of life.

While many religions include meditation as part of their traditions, meditation itself is *not* a religion, and you don't need to be a follower of or convert to any religion to practice basic mindfulness meditation.

As more people learn about the benefits of meditation, the opportunities to learn and practice are becoming more widely available. The meditation in this book is simple, introducing the concept of a steady focus on something like breathing or other sensations in the body.

The beauty of meditation is that it's easy to practice. You can do it from anywhere without special equipment, specific postures or clothes, music or chanting, incense, or any of the other things people often associate with meditation.

Mindfulness meditation can be as simple as two steps: 1) be still and breathe, and 2) notice that you are breathing. Doing these two steps can feel hard at first. Once you're able to focus for even one or two breaths, consider that a win that you can celebrate. As you gain experience, you can keep it simple, or you can go deeper. Most communities have local meditation support groups and courses for further study.

The Benefits of Mindfulness Meditation

There are many benefits of meditation. Scientific studies have shown that with regular practice, mindfulness meditation reduces stress in the short term and provides a long-term stress buffer effect. This means that in the face of your most common daily stressors, you won't react as quickly or strongly. You're better able to choose and control your response.

Many studies show, not surprisingly, that by reducing stress through mindfulness meditation, the many effects of chronic stress on the body are also reduced. Meaning, immune and endocrine measures of inflammation and stress are significantly lower in those who practice mindfulness-based stress reduction (MBSR).[1]

A 2014 meta-analysis of over six hundred research papers found that meditation is more effective than most alternative treatments for anxiety, and that results were directly correlated with the level of stress and anxiety.[2] This means that the more stressed or anxious you are, the better it works.

One randomized control study looked at the effect of using MBSR on health care professionals. The results showed reduced stress and an increase in quality of life and self-compassion among the study participants.[3] In other words, work-related stress can be controlled through meditation.

Another benefit of mindfulness meditation is how it helps you become aware of how you feel, your surroundings, and the choices you have. A 2012 study shows the practice of mindfulness meditation allows the brain to process more creatively. "The authors conclude that mindfulness meditation reduces cognitive rigidity via the tendency to be 'blinded' by experience. Results are discussed in light of the benefits of mindfulness practice regarding a reduced tendency to overlook novel and adaptive ways of responding due to past experience, both in and out of the clinical setting."[4] This means you can stop reacting mindlessly to a familiar situation and use your creative brain to find a better response.

By practicing meditation regularly, you train your brain to maintain focus, thus lengthening your attention span. A longer attention span means you can stay on task longer and, with practice, notice when you're not on task. Further, you develop a greater ability to reorient back to the task if you've wandered off course. This is a significant benefit in the age of attention deficit.[5]

A study of human resource workers showed that "[T]he meditation group reported lower levels of stress and showed better memory for the tasks they had performed; they also switched tasks less often and remained focused on tasks longer."[6]

Other studies have shown meditation helps to reduce age-related memory loss, increase positive feelings and actions toward the self and others, may help fight addictions by increasing self-control and self-awareness of triggers for addictive behaviors, and decrease blood pressure. Another huge benefit of mindfulness meditation is improved sleep.

Most of my clients initially complain of some type of sleep disorder, and statistics show that almost half of the population suffers from lack of sleep. In a study of the effect of meditation on sleep, participants who meditated fell asleep sooner and stayed asleep longer, compared to those who didn't meditate. This alone makes it worth taking the time to practice.[7]

Another benefit of meditation is pain control. Meditators reported less sensitivity to pain and showed increased activity in the brain centers known to control pain.[8]

This list is just a sample of the many proven benefits of a meditation practice. Since you know how helpful it can be for so many things, now is a great time to give it a try. You've already practiced a type of mindfulness meditation earlier in this book, but you might not have realized it. Remember the breathing techniques in Chapter 3? Those are considered examples of mindfulness meditation because you're focusing on your breath and how it feels in your body. Congratulations on the meditation practice you didn't know you have! Now you can go back and practice those exercises with a different mindset.

If you'd like to take your solo meditation practice further, there are several good, free meditation apps for Android and iPhone such as Insight Timer, Headspace, and Stop, Breathe & Think. If you still consider yourself a meditation skeptic, check out 10% Happier created specifically for the skeptic. You can also find other apps that require a fee to access. For group practice, check with local yoga studios or Meetup groups in your area. There are even churches and YMCAs that offer meditation classes.

If you're experiencing resistance to trying mindfulness meditation, I recommend you take a breath and do some EFT Tapping on what you're feeling and where you're feeling it in your body. Meditation has so many benefits, and it's worth discovering how to release any negative energy around trying it.

BONUS - THE PERSONAL PEACE PROCEDURE

Personal Peace. It's a great goal to have, and by using the simple yet powerful methods you've learned so far (breathing, celebrating wins, EFT Tapping, and mindfulness meditation), Personal Peace is available to you with daily practice.

EFT founder Gary Craig created the Personal Peace Procedure to help clear out years and years of accumulated small (and not so small) negative issues you haven't dealt with yet. If you have enough of these issues, they build up and create blockages in the body's energy system. It's time for some cleaning and clearing.

A systematic approach is helpful when starting your Personal Peace journey. Since each issue or event contributes to current energy imbalances and other problems, it's important to address them all. I recommend you make a list.

You can dedicate a section in your tapping notebook or journal for your list, or use a special notebook dedicated to this Personal Peace Procedure. If you prefer electronic versions, start a spreadsheet. Regardless of your method, start a list of every annoying or bothersome issue from your past. Since this might feel daunting, begin with listing one or two things. Ultimately, your list might have fifty, one hundred, or even two hundred items. That's normal. Understand that your list won't be created or cleared in one day. However, if you tap on one issue each day, you'll have cleared your list within a few months or so. How exciting is it to think you could release negative emotions associated with so many annoying reminders from the past just by tapping a little each day?

You can add to your list when something else comes to mind, or as new memories surface while you're tapping. Many find it easiest to start a list by noting childhood issues. As you write, be concise and specific in your description. You don't want to make the issue too big or too general, or you'll miss clearing the subtle hidden details. So, keep them short, such as a one- to three-minute episode with a beginning, a middle, and an end, as well as defined characters. Give each issue a descriptive title or name, like "That time when I was six, and my Mom said I couldn't spend the night with my friend!"

As you compile your list, put a number next to each issue from 0 to 10 to indicate your current intensity of emotion around it. You may want to prioritize and tackle some of the more intense issues first or rotate between higher intensity and lower intensity issues. You might set a goal of tapping each day on a specific number of issues. Follow your instincts to find a method that works best for you.

After clearing a few highly charged issues, or after clearing a certain number of events, you can go back through your list and note which emotional intensities need to be updated.

Thanks to the Generalization Effect in EFT, as you tap through and resolve issues, other issues may become less intense. I love that about Tapping! Because you can make great progress quickly, you should continue adding to and clearing events on your list until you can get through almost all of them, or even finish the list. It can be tempting to stop when you start feeling a little better, but keep going. Don't leave anything under the rug. It is *so* worth it.

As you clear out your old energy disruptions, you'll begin to notice subtle and sometimes even dramatic positive changes in your life. You may start sleeping better, eating healthier, feeling more confident, noticing less stress, and experiencing less frustration at home and at work. You might even be smiling and feeling thankful more often! EFT can help you in so many ways if you just remember to tap every single day.

That was a ton of information, so here's a quick summary to get you started on your Personal Peace Procedure:

1. Start a list of specific bothersome issues or events from your past.
2. Rank the intensity of your emotions about each event from 0 to 10.
3. Tap on one or more events each day.
4. Review the list of events and their intensities periodically as you progress.
5. Notice the positive changes in your life.
6. Celebrate!

Remember: It's important to contact a professional if things feel too big for you, whether it be a physician, psychologist, psychiatrist, or certified EFT coach. Never discontinue your current medications without first consulting your doctor.

Ways to Strengthen Your Stress-Relief Skills

- Continue your daily breathing practices, especially during stressful times.
- Continue celebrating and documenting your daily wins.
- Listen to the guided relaxation audios when you need a break.
- Begin your Personal Peace journey by starting your list of past issues that still hold a charge for you, noting the intensity of each.
- Use EFT Tapping daily! Work on your list in a systematic way to address one or more issues each day.
- Review the "How to be the Calm in the Storm" bonus section in the previous chapter to make sure you're comfortable with the process so that when the next crisis hits, you're ready. Don't forget to customize this process for yourself. You're doing a great job of building your custom stress-relief toolbox one tool at a time.
- Look in the mirror and tell yourself "I've got this!"

Journaling Your Experience

Have you given yourself the gift of listening to the seven-minute guided relaxation audio in your Relax, Tap, and Rest Kit? If so, describe any benefits you noticed. These may change over time, so note your first reactions here for later reference.

_____

_____

_____

_____

_____

_____

_____

_____

_____

_____

_____

_____

_____

_____

_____

_____

_____

_____

_____

_____

_____

_____

_____

_____

_____

_____

_____

What thoughts are you having about starting the Personal Peace Procedure?

_____

_____

_____

_____

_____

_____

_____

_____

_____

_____

_____

_____

If you're feeling resistance to starting this process, tap about the resistance. Describe what comes up about your resistance below.

_____

_____

_____

_____

_____

_____

_____

_____

_____

_____

_____

_____

If you've started your Personal Peace Procedure, what positive changes are you seeing and feeling in your life?

_____

_____

_____

_____

_____

_____

_____

_____

_____

_____

_____

Describe how it feels when you look in the mirror and tell yourself "I've got this!" I hope it feels great and true! But if you notice any resistance to looking yourself in the eye and saying this, try tapping about what you feel.

_____

_____

_____

_____

_____

_____

_____

_____

_____

_____

_____

Chapter 9

Discover Profound Rest

You'll continue to build and deepen your guided relaxation and meditation tools and be introduced to a new method that provides the benefits of deep sleep in this chapter. All you have to do is lie comfortably still and listen to a twenty-five-minute guided relaxation session. With practice, you'll be able to relax deeply just by listening to this powerful meditation. And you'll continue to enjoy feeling well-rested and well-resourced, no matter what demands are put on your time.

INTRODUCTION TO YOGA NIDRA

Yoga nidra is a guided meditation that provides a systematic, progressive awareness of the breath and the body, which leads to profoundly deep rest and calm. I call it a power nap. Everyone, including children as young as three, can benefit from a guided yoga nidra session.

Guided yoga nidra sessions can be as short as five minutes or as long as sixty minutes or more, so you can choose a length based on the time you have available. It's offered at different yoga studios or as audios, which you can listen to online or even download. You don't need to practice yoga to practice yoga nidra, as it involves no movements at all.

Yoga nidra means "yogic sleep," and it's described as the deepest possible state of relaxation while still remaining conscious. You may feel like you're drifting in and out of sleep, but your subconscious still hears the words as you are guided into this deep state of rest.

A yoga nidra session can be just as restorative as sleep. Used prior to your sleep time, it allows for a gentle slowing down and focusing of your mind, helping you to drift off more easily when you finish the session. All you need to do is get comfortable in your bed and listen to a guided session, using earphones if you like. As long as you're comfortable and able to be still, you'll benefit from this practice. More than once, I've awakened with the earphones still in my ears after an especially relaxing session!

BENEFITS OF YOGA NIDRA

1. Less stress! Yoga nidra calms, quiets, and brings clarity to the mind and body and allows for full-body relaxation. It's even better than a typical mindfulness meditation for reducing stress. By giving the mind a continual moving focus during the progressive body and breath scan, the nervous system calms, and we reduce our stress levels. Studies over the past four decades by Dr. Richard Miller, Rod Stryker, and many others have shown that a yoga nidra practice is beneficial for stress and post-traumatic stress disorder (PTSD). As Rod Stryker points out, "We live in a chronically exhausted, overstimulated world."[1] Yoga nidra helps relieve the daily stress we face.

2. More sleep! A 2016 randomized controlled study of twenty-nine individuals with sleep disorders showed that the yoga nidra meditation group experienced a significantly longer time asleep than the two control groups.[2] Easing into sleep after a yoga nidra session is something you need to experience to fully understand. You'll feel comforted and relaxed as you drift off more easily, and practicing yoga nidra also helps you fall back to sleep if you wake up in the middle of the night. Overcoming insomnia is a good thing.

3. A 2011 randomized controlled trial of one hundred fifty women showed that both anxiety and depression decreased significantly in the group that practiced yoga nidra. In addition, positive well-being, general health, and vitality improved significantly after six months of yoga nidra practice when compared with the control group who did not practice yoga nidra.[3]

4. A yoga nidra practice allows increased self-awareness. This practice brings you to a relaxed state, which can help you calmly recognize and acknowledge old stress response habits

and create more helpful responses to those triggers. Awareness is the important first step. Making a better choice then becomes possible. We create new and better habits when we're aware of the old ones.

5. A regular practice of yoga nidra allows you to carry the calm and relaxed feeling you find during your practice back into your daily life, so your confident, creative brain can do its best. It allows you to feel more connected to self and others, which reduces stress by decreasing feelings of loneliness and separation.

PRACTICE YOGA NIDRA

The best way to understand the benefits of yoga nidra is to try it. You will find a free twenty-five-minute guided yoga nidra audio included in your Relax, Tap, and Rest Kit by signing up at https://FromStressed-ToCalm.com/bookbonus/.

During this practice, you'll recline in a comfortable position, fully supported so you can rest without moving. You'll be gently guided through setting an intention for your session. This intention could be a heartfelt desire you have and would like to see as truth, for yourself or for someone else. For example, learning to react to stress in a healthier way might be a heartfelt desire to set if that feels right for you. Or, think about anything you'd like to achieve. Think Big!

Then you'll be guided through a brief awareness of the breath, followed by focusing awareness on individual parts of the head and body. You'll explore opposites of sensations, which definitely gives the busy mind something to focus on. As the meditation nears its end, you'll be guided to gently wake the body. You'll also revisit and reaffirm your intention before you finish. This process is an amazing gift to yourself. It will reduce your stress, which will lead to feelings of complete relaxation, joy, well-being, connection, and peace.

You can find additional free yoga nidra practices on the meditation apps mentioned in the previous chapter. Try practices from several different teachers to experience a range of lengths, voices, sounds, and areas of concentration. Choose several you like and set up a regular practice, perhaps weekly. I know your time is limited, but I believe once you've tried yoga nidra a few times, you'll agree that it deserves to be a priority.

Journaling Your Experience

Have you given yourself the gift of listening to the twenty-five-minute guided yoga nidra audio in your Relax, Tap, and Rest Kit? If so, describe your reaction to this experience. (If not, notice if you have any resistance to giving yourself that time, and tap on that!)

_____

_____

_____

_____

_____

_____

_____

_____

_____

_____

_____

_____

_____

_____

_____

_____

_____

_____

_____

_____

_____

_____

_____

_____

_____

_____

Chapter 10

Rediscover Your Brilliance

Several strategic methods that increase and enhance your energy are provided in this chapter. You'll learn how to reignite your inner spark to rediscover your brilliant self. You'll learn powerful techniques to first recognize, and then begin to set, boundaries that others will understand and respect, and you'll learn tactful ways of saying "no" that will become easier with practice.

But first let me ask: how is your breathing practice going? Has a slow, comfortably deep breath become your automatic response in a stressful moment? Are you celebrating and writing down your wins each day? How about EFT Tapping? I know this technique can be challenging at first to find space and time to practice, but only five minutes each day can make a world of difference in managing stress and overwhelm. We'll use tapping again in this chapter to help us learn to set boundaries and more easily say "no." I hope you're giving yourself the gift of self-care by practicing your stress relief techniques daily.

Setting Boundaries

In order to interact with the world in a positive way, you need to feel in control of life, which is why it's important to recognize, understand, and be able to calmly set your boundaries—before someone crosses one inadvertently.

Do you know what your boundaries are? Have you experienced a boundary-crossing that left you shocked and angry? Do you go into fight, flight, or worse, freeze mode where you can't react, or even speak? Do you feel angry and resentful later, once you've had time to unfreeze, think, and create scenarios you wish could have happened instead? If this describes you, wouldn't it be great to break that cycle?

When thinking specifically of boundaries at work, it can be a powerful exercise to identify what boundaries you already have. For example, do you have a boundary about how many extra hours you're willing to work on a shift, in a day, or in a week? As quoted often from an unknown author: "True strength is found in standing firm yet bending gently." Flexibility can be beneficial to all when appropriate, but not to the extent that you're working so many hours it's impacting your health or your personal life.

What about physical space? If you work in a shared space with others, you may have boundaries about your workspace, your chair, where you put your paperwork or your belongings. What other boundaries might you have or need in your specific work situation? What makes you feel uncomfortable or stressed at work that could be made better by setting a boundary you need?

Setting boundaries is an important component of core emotional health and well-being because it allows you to maintain healthy and productive working relationships on your terms. It's important to note that setting boundaries isn't about avoiding responsibilities, obligations, or rules.

You can learn to more easily recognize and set healthy boundaries by using EFT Tapping to clear negative emotions that arise when someone crosses a boundary. These negative emotions are what get in the way of you calmly setting boundaries. When you tap to clear these negative emotions, you're able to see there's an easier way to set boundaries.

Setting Boundaries Practice

Bring to mind a time when someone crossed a boundary. For this first practice, keep it small, nothing that will trigger a big reaction. Now imagine this person is standing right in front of you, and you could ask them or tell them something about the incident.

- As you imagine doing this, *what emotion comes up*? Is it anger, fear, hurt, resentment, guilt, curiosity, or something else? It may be more than one emotion, but what is the one you notice *first*? Name that emotion.
- *Where do you feel that* emotion in your body? What does it feel like? How big is it? Does it have a color? Describe that feeling in your body and use those exact words when you tap.
- On a scale of *0 to 10*, how intense is that feeling in your body at this moment? Write that number down as your starting point.
- *Begin tapping* on the *side of the hand* point as you say your setup statement. Be as specific as you can with what you feel in your body. Here is an example to help you get started: "Even though I feel this anger and have this tightness in my chest at about an 8 when I think about this incident, I completely accept myself and how I feel." Repeat the setup statement three times while tapping on the *side of the hand* point, using words that seem best for your situation.
- Continue tapping through the other eight tapping points while repeating a reminder phrase, such as "This tightness in my chest," or, "All this anger," at each point.

After one round of tapping through all the points, take a slow breath and do a quick check-in. How intense is that feeling in your body now on a scale of 0 to 10? Compare this with your original number. If it's still above a 3, continue tapping on this feeling using very specific words until it's a 3 or below. Remember that as you tap, other memories or emotions about the incident may come up, or the feeling in your body may change locations. This is all normal. Change your words to match what you're feeling and where you're feeling it.

Now that your intensity is a 3 or below, it's time to test your work. Testing is a very important part of getting lasting benefits from EFT

Tapping. Imagine, again, this person standing in front of you. You're asking or telling them something about the incident. Is there any change in your intensity? If your intensity goes up again, tap another round or two to get it back down to 3 or below.

Once the first physical and emotional sensations have been released, notice what else comes up. Begin tapping on each emotion you're feeling and where you feel it in your body, one at a time, until that entire incident has no remaining emotional charge.

As mentioned earlier, thanks to the Generalization Effect with EFT Tapping, you'll likely not need to tap on every single emotion because as you tap down the intensity of one or two emotions, the intensity of the other emotions may decrease as well. Keep checking in and tapping as needed.

Did you remember any other boundary incidents? Were you reminded of an earlier time when a similar incident happened? Write it down so you can tap on it, either right away or later. When you think about that incident, notice what you feel, where you feel it, rate the intensity, and tap.

By tapping in this way, you're removing the emotional blockages about this one incident. And more importantly, you're rewiring your brain's habit of reacting in a certain way around this type of incident, making it less likely to trigger you or make you freeze again. Once you clear and release the negative emotions associated with an incident or a particular person, it's much easier to set healthy boundaries with that person or others in a similar situation. If you stay calm and aware, you can communicate rationally and set the boundaries you need. As with everything else, it really does get easier with practice.

Having Trouble Setting a Boundary?

Tapping really helps with this as well. When you think about setting a boundary, notice what feelings come up. It may be fear of someone's reaction, a feeling of guilt, or feeling you're not good enough or don't deserve to have this boundary. Once you identify the emotion, notice where you feel it in your body, what that looks like, and how intense it is from 0 to 10. Use descriptive and specific words. At the *end* of your setup statement, try using this powerful permission: "I give myself permission to set this healthy boundary."

The technique of imagining the person in front of you is very helpful for other reasons as well. In particular,

- you get a chance to practice what you'd say to them before it happens, and
- you can imagine their response when you make a request for the boundary you need, so you're better prepared to respond.

Tap on any reaction you might have to their possible responses, so you're ready for anything. You could even have a friend role-play with you to practice what you'd like to say to that person until you're comfortable.

Setting boundaries is a powerful and healthy way of reducing stress and helping you feel safe, in control, and calm both at work and at home. When you're able to recognize and set boundaries, you invite more freedom and joy into your life. You have more energy, which allows you to do more of the things you truly enjoy. I encourage you to explore what boundaries you'd like to set for a more relaxing and fulfilling life and a more creative and brilliant you.

Ten Ways to Say "No" with Ease

Are you a people pleaser? Are you always saying "yes" when you don't have the time or the interest in what's being asked of you? Do you often put the needs of others before your own?

How would it feel if you could say "no" in a way that doesn't hurt anyone's feelings or burn bridges? What if you could reduce the stress in your life and free up a little time on your calendar by saying that one little word—"no"? With practice, courage, calming breaths, and EFT Tapping, you can do this!

Here are just a few ways to say "no."

1. *"I appreciate your asking, but I can't."* If you know that it's not something you can or want to do, let them know by declining right then. This statement is simple, direct, easy to remember, and polite. No long explanation is needed. You're doing them a favor by letting them know right away so they can make other arrangements. You're doing yourself a favor by not letting the request drag on when you know already that you can't or don't want to do it.

2. *"Let me think about that,"* or *"Can I get back to you?"* If it's something you might be willing to do, you can decide after you've had a little time on your own to think. This answer is easier than a quick "no." As soon as you decide, let them know, so it's not looming over you and creating added stress.

3. *"Thanks, but that doesn't work for me,"* is simple and easy. No explanation needed.

4. *"Oh, I wish I could."* I love this one. You don't need to follow up with an excuse. Instead, if you feel the need to say more, you can follow up with a polite, *"but thanks for asking,"* or, *"maybe next time,"* if either of those are true.

5. *"I can't help you this time, but maybe I can help you find someone else who can."* If you have an idea of someone else who could help, or you know of an alternate solution, this works nicely. But if you don't know of someone else, don't add to your stress and your to-do list by saying you do!

6. *"Here's what will work for me,"* or *"Here's what I can do."* Perhaps you have time and would like to help, but can't do everything they want exactly when they want it. You can be specific about what you *can* do with this compromise statement.

7. *"I can't help you right now, but I'll let you know when I have time."* This is a polite way of saying "no" without shutting the door entirely. And of course, use this only if you're willing to keep that door open! Otherwise, you're prolonging the agony, guilt, and stress.

8. *"I'm focusing my time on . . . right now, so I have to say 'no' for now."* Be honest and share what you're focusing on if you want to continue the conversation.

9. *"I'm over-extended right now, and I can't take on any more commitments."* Probably true, right? So, you can say this honestly and with confidence. If it makes you feel better, you can always add, *"But thanks for asking."*

10. *"It's nice of you to think of me, but I really can't help out this time."* Very simple and polite.

Try practicing these statements in front of a mirror until they start to feel natural. Remember that you're practicing self-care when you say "no" to something that isn't a good fit for you. Begin noticing when you say "yes" out of habit. Awareness is a big step.

After you've said "no," be ready to stand your ground, especially if people know you normally always say "yes." They may ask more than once. A simple *"As I mentioned . . ."* will remind them you've already answered. Don't let the guilt monster get the better of you.

With practice, saying "no" gets easier, reduces your stress, builds self-confidence, and gives you more energy for what you love to do. You'll discover a new sense of control and power over your life, and more freedom to say "yes" to things you enjoy.

JOURNALING YOUR EXPERIENCE

Hopefully, after reading this chapter you've been able to practice the methods suggested, and you've been able to tap when facing difficulties. Have you been able to set a new boundary when you discovered you needed to? If so, describe here how that felt. If not, what do you think you might need to be able to try?

_____

_____

_____

_____

_____

_____

_____

_____

_____

_____

_____

_____

_____

_____

_____

_____

_____

_____

_____

_____

_____

_____

_____

_____

Have you used any of the ten ways to say "no" yet? Which ones do you think will work best for you?

_____

_____

_____

_____

_____

_____

_____

_____

_____

_____

_____

_____

_____

_____

_____

_____

_____

_____

_____

_____

_____

_____

_____

_____

_____

_____

_____

_____

_____

Chapter 11

Discover Confidence

Definitions of confidence, especially regarding self-confidence, can make us feel good just reading them. Here are a few I especially like:

- A feeling of self-assurance arising from your appreciation of your abilities or qualities.
- A feeling or consciousness of your powers.
- A feeling or belief you can do something well or succeed at something.
- A feeling that allows you to stand up for yourself and your beliefs.

The last one rings true as it applies to setting healthy boundaries as discussed in the previous chapter.

Confidence seems to come and go for many people, depending on the day, the situation, or the people involved. Like most things, confidence can become stronger and second nature for you when you consciously practice feeling better about yourself, and when you intentionally notice and appreciate your own abilities. Because everyone has their strengths, sometimes it's best to leave certain tasks in the hands of an expert. When you have confidence, you're able to let go of those tasks, knowing they'll be done well.

Confidence Boosters

Just like the other tools and techniques you've learned already, when you practice feeling confident, your confidence grows. So, let's consider ways of boosting your confidence with quotes sprinkled in to inspire you toward greatness.

Choose the ones that work best for you and leave the rest for now. They may work better at another time. The point is to create a custom blend of techniques that works best for *you*, so you replace self-criticism with self-confidence and maintain a sense of calm and balance going forward, no matter what your days bring.

"Each time we face our fear, we gain strength, courage, and confidence in the doing."

~ *Theodore Roosevelt*

---

1. *Smile*. I hope you've been practicing this since Chapter 4! This one is *so* easy, and research shows it works to reduce stress and lower the heart rate, which leads to feeling calmer and more confident. Try it now as you're reading this. It's a quick and easy way to feel more self-confident and to help those around you to see you in a more confident light!

"Self-confidence is the most attractive quality a person can have. How can anyone see how great you are, if you can't see it yourself?"

~ *Unknown*

---

2. *Write down your strengths*. This only takes a few minutes, but can make a huge impact on your self-confidence. Start with your top five strengths. Since most people aren't always able to identify their strengths, call a few supportive and honest friends to help you with this task. Their answers and consistency may surprise you. If you have more than five to list, go for it! I recommend putting this list in a place where you'll see it daily. Decorate it, put smiley faces or stickers on it to make your list as special as you are. Celebrate your list.

"With realization of one's own potential and self-confidence in one's ability, one can build a better world."

~ *Dalai Lama[1]*

---

3. *Have awesome posture.* This is an easy fix that takes zero time. I know it sounds like an overused parental reminder, but when you stand or sit up straight, you feel better about yourself. You automatically appear confident and more attractive to others. If you're like me, it will take a little reminding. I have a bad habit of hunching over my laptop. Use your Mad Ninja Awareness Skills here for awesome posture and confidence.

"Don't wait until everything is just right. It will never be perfect. There will always be challenges, obstacles and less than perfect conditions. So what? Get started now. With each step you take, you will grow stronger and stronger, more and more skilled, more and more self-confident and more and more successful."

~ *Mark Victor Hansen*[2]

---

4. *Do one small thing.* Look at your task list for the day. Identify one small thing you can knock out quickly. Do it. Celebrate your achievement and smile. I realize there may be many things on your task list, and only so much time to do them. Rather than getting stuck in that thought and doing them poorly or not at all, choose one with which you know you can be successful. There is nothing like a victory to build confidence. Allow that victory momentum to carry you forward through your day. It's OK to seed your task list with easy wins when you need them. Smile.

"Because one believes in oneself, one doesn't try to convince others. Because one is content with oneself, one doesn't need others' approval. Because one accepts oneself, the whole world accepts him or her."

~ *Lao Tzu*

---

5. *Eat healthy meals and snacks*. Make meals a special time (at work too), even when you're eating alone. As you eat, look away from your devices, be sure you're sitting down, notice what you're eating, and take in your surroundings Additionally, when at home, turn off the television (that can be a stress-relief technique in itself), set a beautiful table, light a candle, and take a moment to feel grateful. Whether at work or at home, by honoring your meal times, your digestive system will thank you. Healthy food makes you feel better and reduces stress. When you feel better, you'll feel more confident. It's as easy as that.

"Noble and great. Courageous and determined. Faithful and fearless. That is who you are and who you have always been. And understanding it can change your life, because this knowledge carries a confidence that cannot be duplicated any other way."

~ Sheri L. Dew[3]

---

6. *Get some sleep*. Along the same self-care path, make sure you're getting plenty of sleep. I know that stress, or just life, can keep you awake or disturb your sleep. You can set yourself up for more restful sleep if you set a consistent time to turn off or at least silence all electronic devices and consciously wind down before going to sleep. This is the perfect time to write in your Celebrating Wins notebook to help you find sleep with a grateful heart. You can also practice smiling, do one of the breathing exercises, or practice EFT Tapping on one or two items. You can use a Stealth Technique as you lie back with your eyes closed to help you drift off peacefully.

"One important key to success is self-confidence. An important key to self-confidence is preparation."

~ Arthur Ashe[4]

---

7. *Dress it up.* Wear comfortable clothes that make you feel good about how you look. When you feel good about what you're wearing, you stand taller (see number three above), move more easily, and exude confidence. You don't need to spend a fortune on clothes to look and feel great. You can do that by limiting your wardrobe to just the good stuff, your favorites, the things you absolutely love. By mixing and matching quality separates, your life becomes easier. Investigate capsule wardrobe suggestions to save time by making the what to wear decision a breeze.

"Have confidence that if you have done a little thing well, you can do a bigger thing well too."

~ David Storey[5]

---

8. *Find joy daily.* Think about the things you enjoy. Make a plan, set a goal, do whatever it takes to *do one thing* you enjoy doing *each day*. Doing this will become easier with practice. It can be as simple as spending five minutes outdoors, if that's what makes you happy. Spend quality downtime with someone you care about and be fully present. Eat the occasional dessert. Literally stop to smell the rose. What makes you happy? Do that . . . *today*. You do deserve it. (And if that last statement isn't true for you, can you tap on it?)

"Don't you dare, for one more second, surround yourself with people who are not aware of the greatness that you are."

~ Jo Blackwell-Preston[6]

---

9. *Work it out.* Take the stairs. Park far away from entrances. Walk. Bike. Run. Go to the gym. Take a hike. Go for a swim. Practice yoga. Play soccer. Go paddling. Dance. Go skiing. You get the idea. Move daily. Move your body in different ways. Move

enough to sweat three times each week. Your health will improve, you'll look and feel better, and your clothes will look and feel better on you giving you more confidence!

> *"Wouldn't it be powerful if you fell in love with yourself so deeply that you would do just about anything if you knew it would make you happy? This is precisely how much life loves you and wants you to nurture yourself. The deeper you love yourself, the more the universe will affirm your worth. Then you can enjoy a lifelong love affair that brings you the richest fulfillment from inside out."*
>
> ~ Alan Cohen[7]

10. *Speak with confidence.* Speak slowly. Speak loud enough that you're easily heard. Make eye contact whether you're speaking to one person or to a group. These are all the marks of someone in authority. If it feels awkward at first, practice a few times in the mirror to become more comfortable. Practice with friends and then take it into the world.

> *"Our deepest fear is not that we are inadequate. Our deepest fear is that we are powerful beyond measure. It is our light, not our darkness that most frightens us. We ask ourselves, 'Who am I to be brilliant, gorgeous, talented, fabulous?' Actually, who are you not to be? You are a child of God. Your playing small does not serve the world. There is nothing enlightened about shrinking so that other people won't feel insecure around you. We are all meant to shine, as children do. And as we let our own light shine, we unconsciously give other people permission to do the same. As we are liberated from our own fear, our presence automatically liberates others."*
>
> ~ Marianne Williamson[8]

Bonus Confidence Booster

You can tap away fears to uncover your confidence. If fear of failure is keeping you from feeling confident about trying something, you can use EFT Tapping to help you be your best self. Everyone experiences fear sometimes, but successful people don't let it stop them. One of my mentors uses the phrase "Fail forward." Failure can be an amazing teacher when you learn from it and use that knowledge to continue moving forward.

Use EFT Tapping to release the fear. Start by investigating the fear. What are you feeling, where are you feeling it in your body, and how intense is it right now? Tap as many rounds as you need to reduce the intensity and then notice how you feel. See if you can release the fear enough to move forward any amount. Tap early, tap often, and celebrate your successes!

"Whether you think you can or think you can't, you are right."

~ Henry Ford[9]

CHECKING IN

- How is your breathing practice going? Which one or two are you using most often? It's good to know what works for you but definitely go back and try the others when you have time. Things change. People change.

- Are you writing down or typing up your wins each day? Try keeping your wins journal up to date daily as you go forward.

- How about EFT Tapping? Are you comfortable with the Basic Recipe and the Stealth Techniques? Are you working on your Personal Peace Procedure list?

- Were you able to notice where you might need a boundary? Any progress on tapping about boundary emotions from past incidents?

- What tools are working best for you overall?

- Review the Confidence Boosters. Do any of these suggestions sound easy to implement? Start with adding one or two to your toolbox until they become a habit, and then you can add others that look easy.

Take a little time to review and optimize your stress-relief toolbox, so you're prepared for any occasion. With a commitment to a continued regular use of these self-care tools, you'll experience stress relief and a calmer, happier you.

JOURNALING YOUR EXPERIENCE

From the list of Confidence Boosters in this chapter, which one will you try first? Describe how it feels to plan this action. Tap for any resistance. Go! You can do this! (And once you've tried one, choose the next one to try!)

Describe your current stress-relief toolbox. What's the first tool you use when you notice stress? What's your favorite tool and why?

_____

_____

_____

_____

_____

_____

_____

_____

_____

_____

_____

_____

_____

_____

_____

_____

_____

_____

_____

_____

_____

_____

_____

_____

_____

_____

Chapter 12

Go-To Stress-Relief Tools

Do you find that at times you're so stressed that your rational thinking brain leaves the building and you freeze? This chapter includes a list of quick solutions and tools you can use in different situations to unfreeze, so you can think clearly and efficiently again. Some of these have already been discussed in previous chapters, but they're worth repeating here.

The list below is just to get you started. Add to your list when you discover new techniques that work for you. Experiment with techniques that use the different senses until you find the combination that works best. Remember, you're a dynamic being whose needs may change over time, so revisit the list occasionally to make sure it's still serving you well.

Practice these tools as often as you can so they become second nature to you. Rather than waiting for a stressful moment to remember a tool that will help you find calm, use them multiple times each day so you can call them up easily when you need them. Try them all to find the ones that feel best to you.

Breathe. Take five slow, comfortably deep, focused breaths. If you can stop and be still for a minute, that's even better, but do become aware of your breathing. If you like, use your favorite breathing practice from Chapter 3 for a few minutes.

Tap. Begin tapping on the *side of the hand*, any of the points on the upper body, or tap or hold the finger points. Do what seems right for you at that moment. No words are needed to start tapping. Just tap gently. Let the calming "all is well" signal get to your brain, so you can think clearly again. Words may or may not come, and either way, it's fine. Just tap.

Take a break. Get outside if possible, but even walking to the restroom and back can help. Walk up and down a flight of stairs if there are any available. Any exercise will help reduce stress and make you feel better.

<u>*Drink a glass of water*</u>. Dehydration can cause you to feel stressed and irritable. Drinking water also has the added benefit of keeping you from mindlessly eating comfort food. Often when you think you're hungry, you're just thirsty. Herbal teas can be calming as well. Make sure you're not avoiding liquids so you don't have to use the restroom, please. Take time to care for you.

Have a small, healthy snack. Sometimes you may need a little blood sugar boost to think more clearly, find a better mood, and feel more in control. Choose with awareness. Hummus + celery
Apples + peanut butter (low glycemic index) + wine

Think a happy thought. Break the stress cycle by taking a quick mental break. Bring to mind a <u>beautiful memory</u>, story, or the <u>image of a loved one to bring a smile to your face</u>. Keep it simple. Let it be something or someone you can recall instantly when you need it. Let your happy thoughts turn your stressful moment around. Keep a picture with you, or in your workspace, of a loved one or a place that feels like an escape for you.

Find the good. In every situation, no matter how stressful, there's something you can find for which you can be grateful. Look around, find something, and say to yourself, or even out loud, "thank you." It can be the tiniest of things, but it can be powerful enough to lift you up. Your heart will soften, and you may even smile. Whenever I see a beautiful sunrise or sunset, I often say "thank you" with my out loud voice. I find doing this makes the experience even better and helps me see more good things.

Stretch. Stand up, reach overhead, and then reach out to the sides. Let your face and neck relax. Relax your arms down again. Slowly and gently look up and then down once or twice. You can twist from the waist side to side a few times to get the energy flowing. While sitting, you can rotate at the ankle several times, pointing and flexing. Stretch in any way that works for you where you are.

Tune in. If you have the time and the situation allows for it, listen to a short, guided relaxation or meditation. Take five minutes to close your eyes, be still, focus inward, and breathe slowly and deeply.

Listen. If music helps bring you to a calmer place, keep a device for listening nearby with a selection of music that makes you happy. While this isn't always possible at work, you can plan your selections for your commute rather than getting spun up with the news and those never-ending adrenaline-driven advertisements on the radio.

Calming scents. Keep a bottle or two of calming essential oils, such as lavender, chamomile, or rose oils, nearby to help release stress. Just open and enjoy. Light a scented candle at home. (Be considerate of others who may be overly sensitive or allergic to strong scents.)

Go soak. Plan time to soak in a warm or cool bath. You might want music or bath oils to make it a special treat. The planning and antici-pation of a quiet time of self-care can get you through stressful times.

Pets. If you have a pet, it's a win-win to go scratch or brush them. They love it, and this calms you as well.

Call a friend. Sometimes talking about things with someone can help. Connect with your friend even if you're not ready to talk about a stressful situation. Just the sense of connection and community can be grounding and supportive.

Enjoy the process of experimenting with different ways to relieve stress. If something isn't helpful, there's no need to force it. Not all of these suggestions will work for everyone or in all places, but make an effort to find what works for you and practice, practice, practice.

JOURNALING YOUR EXPERIENCE

What is the first Go-To Stress-Relief Tool you will try? Why that one?
(And once you've tried one, choose the second one!)

_____

_____

_____

_____

_____

_____

_____

_____

_____

_____

_____

_____

_____

_____

_____

_____

_____

_____

_____

_____

_____

_____

_____

_____

_____

_____

_____

_____

Afterword

Congratulations! You now have a collection of tools that can quickly and easily take you to a better place. Celebrate the journey and effort you've made in learning and practicing the different tools in this book.

Here's a quick example of how you can take a few minutes to turn your day around using a combination of these stress-relief tools. Customize these suggestions to suit your situation and needs.

1. *Notice.* When stress starts to take over, it's really important to notice what's happening. Pay attention. You'll use this information later when you tap.
2. *Start breathing* using one of the techniques that will work in the situation. Simply taking five slow, quiet, comfortably deep breaths during a stressful time will start the calming process.
3. Look around and *find one thing* that is good, beautiful, funny, or makes you smile. Remember that for your Celebrating Wins notebook.
4. Find a place to *take a break* that feels comfortable for you to practice breathing and tapping. No need to wait to practice breathing. You can start breathing on the way.
5. *Tap.* Notice how you feel in that moment. Where do you feel it in your body? How intensely? Using the Basic Recipe, tap for one emotion, sensation, or event at a time. If you can't find the words, tap without words. As you calm down, words may come. Tap as long as you are able during your break. Even one round without words will calm you significantly and let your rational brain come back online. You'll make better decisions and feel more confident. That's another win worth celebrating!

6. Remember to *say "no" with confidence* if a request isn't right for you.

All work situations are different. What's possible in one place might not be ideal in another. Personalize these tools to meet your needs and practice them as often as you can—at least daily. Look for ways to incorporate them into your day: bathroom breaks, elevators, stairwells, a quick walk outside are all good options. Before you know it, you'll find yourself starting to breathe as a calming practice "automagically." You'll start noticing more things to celebrate, and you'll get so good at tapping you'll start doing it easily nearly everywhere. You have Stealth Tapping techniques you can practice anywhere, too.

I would *love* to hear from you as to what works for you and what doesn't.

Reach out to me at Terry@FromStressedToCalm.com.

If this book was helpful to you, please consider providing your honest review on Amazon. This will help the book reach more people who need it!

Thank you so much.

Notes

Chapter 2

1. American Institute of Stress: http://www.stress.org
2. If you love a good scientific read about stress and hormones, see this article found on the U.S. National Institutes of Health website: https://www.ncbi.nlm.nih.gov/pmc/articles/PMC3079864/

Chapter 3

1. The Effect of Diaphragmatic Breathing on Attention, Negative Affect and Stress in Healthy Adults: https://www.ncbi.nlm.nih.gov/pmc/articles/PMC5455070/
2. Relaxation techniques: Breath control helps quell errant stress response: https://www.health.harvard.edu/mind-and-mood/relaxation-techniques-breath-control-helps-quell-errant-stress-response
3. Relax, Take a Deep Breath: https://www.psychiatry.org/newsroom/apa-blogs/apa-blog/2017/06/relax-take-a-deep-breath
4. How Breathing Calms Your Brain, And Other Science-Based Benefits Of Controlled Breathing: https://www.forbes.com/sites/daviddisalvo/2017/11/29/how-breathing-calms-your-brain-and-other-science-based-benefits-of-controlled-breathing/#4770e7752221

Chapter 5

1. Gary Craig, founder of EFT, "Gold Standard" EFT Tapping Tutorial. See https://emofree.com/eft-tutorial/eft-tapping-tutorial.html
2. Gary Craig. See https://emofree.com/articles-ideas/general-ideas/tuningin-article.html

Chapter 8

1. For more information, see "A comparison of mindfulness-based stress reduction and an active control in modulation of neurogenic inflammation." (https://www.sciencedirect.com/science/article/pii/S0889159112004758)

2. For more information, see "Effects of the transcendental meditation technique on trait anxiety: a meta-analysis of randomized controlled trials." (https://www.ncbi.nlm.nih.gov/pubmed/24107199)

3. For more information see "Mindfulness-Based Stress Reduction for Health Care Professionals: Results from a Randomized Trial." (http://psycnet.apa.org/record/2005-05099-004)

4. For more information see "Mind the Trap: Mindfulness Practice Reduces Cognitive Rigidity." (http://journals.plos.org/plosone/article?id=10.1371/journal.pone.0036206)

5. For more information see "Mindfulness training modifies subsystems of attention." (https://link.springer.com/article/10.3758/CABN.7.2.109#page-1)

6. For more information see "Initial results from a study of the effects of meditation on multitasking performance." (https://dl.acm.org/citation.cfm?id=1979862)

7. For more information see "The value of mindfulness meditation in the treatment of insomnia." (https://www.ncbi.nlm.nih.gov/pubmed/26390335)

8. For more information see "Brain Mechanisms Supporting Modulation of Pain by Mindfulness Meditation." (https://www.ncbi.nlm.nih.gov/pmc/articles/PMC3090218/)

Chapter 9

1. Rod Stryker, founder of ParaYoga: https://www.parayoga.com/rod-stryker/

2. For more information see "Comparative Effectiveness of Three Occupational Therapy Sleep Interventions: A Randomized

Controlled Study." (https://www.irest.us/sites/default/files/Sleep_Interventions_Study_Pub_16.pdf)

3. For more information see "Impact of *Yoga Nidra* on psychological general wellbeing in patients with menstrual irregularities: A randomized controlled trial." (https://www.ncbi.nlm.nih.gov/pmc/articles/PMC3099097/)

Chapter 11

1. 100 Inspiring Quotes That Will Increase Your Confidence: https://www.inc.com/lolly-daskal/100-inspiring-quotes-that-will-increase-your-confidence.html

2. Ibid

3. Goodreads: https://www.goodreads.com/quotes/104705-noble-and-great-courageous-and-determined-faithful-and-fearless-that

4. 100 Inspiring Quotes That Will Increase Your Confidence: https://www.inc.com/lolly-daskal/100-inspiring-quotes-that-will-increase-your-confidence.html

5. BrainyQuote: https://www.brainyquote.com/quotes/david_storey_164551

6. Goodreads: https://www.goodreads.com/quotes/685077-don-t-you-dare-for-one-second-surround-yourself-with-people

7. 55 Motivational Quotes That Will Inspire You to Believe in Yourself: https://www.inc.com/jeff-haden/55-motivational-quotes-that-will-inspire-you-to-believe-in-yourself.html

8. Goodreads: https://www.goodreads.com/author/quotes/17297.Marianne_Williamson

9. Goodreads: https://www.goodreads.com/quotes/978-whether-you-think-you-can-or-you-think-you-can-t--you-re

Special Gift from Terry

Now that you've read *Rx for RNs*, you're familiar with the tools to help you recognize and manage stress. Hopefully, you're practicing them daily to learn what works best for you in your life.

If you haven't already, I highly recommend that you sign up for the Relax, Tap, and Rest Kit I created to supplement this book:

- a quick seven-minute guided relaxation audio so you can relax even when you don't have much time,
- a concise "How to Tap" video that clearly demonstrates the EFT Tapping process, and
- a twenty-five-minute guided yoga nidra audio, which is a great way to feel fully rested.

Visit https://FromStressedToCalm.com/bookbonus/ to sign up for your Relax, Tap, and Rest Kit. You'll also receive stress management tips and information from me every few weeks. Your information will never be shared, and you can unsubscribe at any time.

The sooner you practice using these simple tools for releasing stress, the sooner you'll start thinking, feeling, and sleeping better.

Here's to you! You've taken care of everyone and everything else. Now it's your turn.

All the Best,

Terry Maluk

About the Author

Terry Maluk is a gifted speaker, author, and stress-relief specialist. A member of the American Holistic Nurses Association, Terry holds a Master of Science degree in Public Health and is also an accredited, certified Emotional Freedom Techniques (EFT Tapping) practitioner and a registered yoga teacher through Yoga Alliance.

Having spent over 15 years in the fast-paced technology field under constant pressure to do more with less while responding to unexpected crises, Terry learned firsthand about the effects of chronic stress. What seemed to be a series of random physical symptoms became an obvious pattern that began impacting her activities and the quality of her life.

Embarking on her own personal quest to understand not only what was happening but *why*, she discovered how chronic stress impacts the mind and body. The connection between stress and physical and emotional symptoms is real. And there are definitely tools we can use to relieve stress and gain control over our lives again.

As Terry learned a variety of time-honored and scientifically proven stress-relief techniques that reduced her own pain and chronic stress, she began to share with others who were experiencing similar stressful situations. This book is based on her hands-on experience working with clients and seeing the life-changing results they received.

Connect with Terry on LinkedIn: https://www.linkedin.com/in/terry-maluk/
Follow Terry on Twitter: @StressedToCalm
Follow Terry on Facebook: https://www.facebook.com/FromStressedToCalm/
Visit Terry at From Stressed to Calm: https://FromStressedToCalm.com

A12

73385157R00076

Made in the USA
Columbia, SC
03 September 2019